The Motivational Approach to Natural Weight Loss

THE MOTIVATIONAL APPROACH TO NATURAL WEIGHT LOSS

Forgetting Diets Forever

Dr. Shana Schenker

iUniverse, Inc.
New York Bloomington Shanghai

The Motivational Approach to Natural Weight Loss

Forgetting Diets Forever

iUniverse books may be ordered through booksellers or by contacting:

iUniverse
1663 Liberty Drive
Bloomington, IN 47403
www.iuniverse.com
1-800-Authors (1-800-288-4677)

Because of the dynamic nature of the Internet, any Web addresses
or links contained in this book may have changed
since publication and may no longer be valid.

You should not undertake any diet/exercise regimen recommended in this book before
consulting your personal physician. Neither the author nor the publisher shall be
responsible or liable for any loss or damage allegedly arising as a consequence of your
use or application of any information or suggestions contained in this book.

ISBN: 978-0-595-46340-4 (pbk)
ISBN: 978-0-595-71242-7 (cloth)
ISBN: 978-0-595-90635-2 (ebk)

Printed in the United States of America

This book is dedicated to my dad, a very special man. He has motivated me to follow every dream I've ever conceived. As a neotenous Octegenarian, he is a phenomenal role model. I admire and respect him immensely. Thank you dad. I love you with all my heart and soul. To my two older brothers, Dean Schenker and Dr. Marc Schenker, two special men, who have set a high standard of excellence, personally and professionally, thank you. I love you with all my heart and soul.

In memory of my mother, a very special woman, who taught me that life should be lived with passion, joy, love, faith, and compassion. She encouraged me to develop my communication gifts and talents, and this book and my other successes are the direct result of her inspiration and motivation. I miss you and love you with all my heart and soul.

CONTENTS

Chapter 1: The Mind 1

Chapter 2: Fears 11

Chapter 3: Goal-Setting 20

Chapter 4: Motivation 26

Chapter 5: Stress 34

Chapter 6: Relaxation Techniques 45

Chapter 7: Hypnosis 68

Chapter 8: Diet 91

Chapter 9: Exercise 113

Chapter 10: Wisdom of the Ages 123

Chapter 11: The Spirit Within 128

Chapter 12: Spirituality 132

Chapter 13: Smile 140

Bibliography 147

Resources 151

This book was inspired by many in the healing arts who understand the true meaning of utilizing the power of the mind to reach our goals. Our greatest asset, our health, can be achieved with the elimination of poor habits, poor choices, and a negative mindset. Extra weight not only puts extra fat on your external body, it also puts extra weight on your internal body, physiologically and psychologically. Remove the weight in both arenas, and you can move forward with agility and grace and open new doors of opportunity in other areas of your life. You will see new vistas, grab life with gusto, and enjoy the present for what it is—a present. Read and enjoy the Baker's Dozen, 13 chapters filled with ingredients to choose that are natural, habit-forming, inspiring, and effective. Some have been around since the ancient Greeks and Egyptians used their wisdom to create health and happiness. The main side effect is habit-forming: a change in your attitude about your capabilities that will empower you with confidence and enthusiasm; seeds to plant, nourish, and handle with self love and self acceptance, to help you grow inward and blossom outward.

I hope you take the challenge. With patience and passion you can reach the winners circle of successful and lasting weight loss. Be the best you were meant to be. The first ingredient, your mindset, is in the first chapter. This is where all success begins, so naturally I want you to begin at the beginning. Enjoy each chapter as if you were creating the greatest meal of your life. This, in reality, is what you will be doing; creating a meal with natural, healthy, delicious ingredients. You will be the shinning star and you will twinkle with a new energy and exuberance that makes you radiate wherever you go. Although Rome wasn't built in a day, you can begin to build your own masterpiece from day one when you understand the importance imparted in the first chapter. Let your mind and body and spirit be open to the new you; you'll be glad you did. Everything ahead of you is natural food for thought. You can add years to your life and life to your years.

I want to be your "Mind-Body-Spirit" Coach. I have worked with determination and dedication to earn my credentials and expertise to write and present this book to you. I have a Masters Degree in Behavioral Therapy, a Ph.D. in Motivational Psychology, and a Doctorate in Clinical Hypnotherapy. I am certified in Weight Loss and Maintenance and have certifications in sports improvement, stress management, and fears and phobias. I continue to train with professionals in the healing arts and personally utilize the tools I write about in this guidebook. I'm available in the 13 chapters, the Baker's Dozen, for you to read, feel, taste and enjoy. I want you to see the passion in my words. Your attitude will change from "I can't, because" to "I can, because." You will be inspired and ready to beat and defeat any past failures, defeats, and battles of the bulge you've encountered in the past. Your new goal will be addressed with a spirit of acceptance of all the reasons that you can. You'll move forward with grace and agility. I want you to succeed, and you can, for the right reasons, for the most important person in the world, and that person is you. Don't ever forget that you have a personal purpose in life. I want you to win at that purpose with a new mind, body, and spirit; your own. It will be healthier and wealthier and wiser because you embraced the words on these pages. So get ready, aim, fire and hire. Aim for the stars. Fire the old coach. Hire me as your new "Mind-Body-Spirit" Coach. Get ready for an exciting, empowering, and exhilarating journey!

CHAPTER 1

▼

THE MIND

The two most important facts known to humankind: the fact that if you fail to control your mind, you will control nothing else, and we were given free choice. Your mind is your temple. Protect it and treat it as you would treat royalty; with honor, respect, and love. You were given willpower for this purpose. Thoughts are things when they're mixed with definitiveness of purpose, persistence, and passion. "Whatever the mind of man can conceive and believe, it can achieve."

Controlling your mind is the result of self-discipline. You either control your mind or it controls you. It's a habit. You accomplish this discipline by keeping it busy with purpose and following a specific plan of action.

There are no limitations to the power of the mind, except those you acknowledge. The way to have a mind-set of unlimited potential is with faith. Napoleon Hill said: "Faith is the head chemist of the mind." Faith is an attitude which we create by giving our subconscious mind instructions and directions in the way of positive affirmations repeated over and over again. These affirmations become a part of our physical reality. We learn by repetition. We develop a habit by repetition. By feeding our mind positive affirmations in a continuous flow of love, desire, belief, expectancy, and a positive mental attitude, our subconscious will propel us to take action and create success in our life. Positive and negative emotions can't exist simultaneously; either you love something or you hate it; either you fear something or you don't fear something; either you accept something or you reject something. Form the healthy habit of enjoying positive thoughts daily.

The five main ingredients of positive emotions are the emotions of faith, desire, enthusiasm, hope, and love. Man can create nothing which he does not first conceive in the form of an impulse of thought. These are at a subconscious level. The subconscious then begins to immediately translate thoughts into their physical equivalent at the conscious level. We are influenced by our five senses; taste, sight, feel, sound, and touch. The more intense and the more senses we use, the more open and eager our subconscious will be to respond in kind.

In his best selling book "Your Best Life Now," Pastor Joel Osteen lists seven steps to living at your full potential:

1. Enlarge your vision.
2. Develop a healthy self-image.
3. Discover the power of your thoughts and words.
4. Let go of the past.
5. Find strength through adversity.
6. Live to give.
7. Choose to be happy.

I will elaborate briefly on each of the seven steps as they apply to your goal of a slimmer and trimmer you.

1. Enlarge your vision. Before you picked up this book, you saw yourself as a one-sided person. A fat person carrying around this baggage called "lard." I want you to change this vision as you read these words so that you now enlarge that vision to see the person you want to be; an attractive person on the inside and an equally attractive person on the outside, sans the "lard." Go ahead. See that new you now.

2. Develop a healthy self-image. If you don't have a positive and healthy image of yourself, how can you expect others to see the you that you were meant to be. There is an energy that is translated from a healthy

self-image into external energy, and it can be exhilarating and exciting, and it must begin with a positive image of yourself.

3. Discover the power of your thoughts and words. Thoughts really do become words and words really do become reality when you add a goal, a plan, faith, belief, and positive expectations. From this moment on, I want you to change your belief to one of positive expectations in the goal before you, permanent weight loss. Don't give me excuses, just do it.

4. Let go of the past. I don't care what you weighed this morning. Now is where I want you to begin anew. It's literally a new moment and you can create fantastic experiences in your life if you realize this powerful concept. Live in the moment and enjoy the present, internalizing numbers 1, 2, and 3 above.

5. Find strength through adversity. If your past attempts at weight loss have left you feeling alone and abandoned and as if the world is against you, especially the temptations of commercials, fast food chain restaurants, and supersize portions, remember that today is a new day because you are reading this book, written by your "Mind-Body-Spirit" Coach, and I am here for you on these pages for the short and long term, 24/7/365.

6. Live to give. Charity begins at home. This is the home of your mind, the most dynamite powerhouse in the world. Use it to the fullest. Give yourself permission to lose weight. Give yourself love during the journey and beyond. Give yourself pats on the back when you reach your sub-goals along this new and great adventure of becoming the new you.

7. Choose to be happy. Yes my friends. We have many choices in life, and the one I want you to concentrate on and accept now is your choice to be happy. I guarantee you that if you will put a smile on your face and a song in your heart, you will see beauty where you never saw beauty before. Life will be brighter, more exciting, and healthier. What a great concept to understand when someone tells you that you look slimmer and trimmer. You can tell them it all began because you chose to be happy. Choose happiness now and choose it tomorrow and the next day and the day after that. See what miracles you can create. You won't be sorry, you'll be happy.

The subconscious mind consists of a field of consciousness, in which every impulse of thought that reaches the conscious mind through any of the five senses is classified and recorded, and from which thoughts may be recalled or withdrawn, just as documents may be taken from a filing cabinet. If it acts first on the dominating desire which has been combined with an emotional feeling such as faith, we are drawing from the right brain, the creative and imaginative, non-analytical side of the brain.

Think of your subconscious mind as a magnet. Like a magnet, we draw in what we think about constantly. Earl Nightengale said it best: "We become what we think about most of the time." If you're constantly thinking positive, joyous, upbeat, happy thoughts, you'll be positive, joyous, upbeat, and happy. Just like a magnet, you'll attract positive, joyous, upbeat, happy people. Our thoughts also affect our emotions. We will feel the way we think. You must think happy thoughts to be happy. The Scriptures say: "Be constantly renewed in the spirit of your mind, having a fresh, mental and spiritual attitude."

We should imbibe the Buddist Concept of "Mindfulness." Being present to what we are doing now. This is the foundation of a holistic approach to success. When we live a conscious life, we connect spiritually with the opportunities of our unique human abilities. We don't turn our back on life. We learn to appreciate the continuing evolution of consciousness, ie. growth. Mindfulness is a discipline we want to practice daily, like any learned habit. Consciousness is a main ingredient to success. The more conscious we are in any situation, for example eating healthfully, the more possibilities we tend to perceive; therefore, the more options we have; therefore, the more powerful we are.

Conversely, the less conscious we are in any situation, the fewer possibilities that occur to us; therefore, the more inflexible are our responses; therefore, the less effective we are. Mindful Consciousness and self esteem are practical and dynamic ingredients and powerful tools for success. Keep them sharp the way a surgeon keeps his tools of the trade sharp and always ready to point, aim, and fire with energy and assertiveness.

In his book, "The Six Pillars of Self Esteem," Dr. Nathaniel Braden speaks about self esteem and writes: "It is confidence in the efficacy of our mind, in our ability to think. It is confidence in our ability to learn, make appropriate choices and decisions, and respond effectively to change. It is also the experience that success, achievement, fulfillment and happiness are right and normal for us."

The Six Pillars of Self Esteem are:

1. The practice of acceptance: This refers to ones willingness to take responsibility for our feelings, thoughts, and actions without denial. You give yourself permission to think your own thoughts, experience your true emotions, and look at your actions without condemnation.

2. The practice of self-responsibility: Realizing that we are the writers of our lives and we have choices, and therefore responsibility to accept our choices.

3. The practice of self-assertiveness: Being true to ourselves when we deal with others. Treating our values and who we truly are with self-respect. The willingness to stand up for ourselves and our ideas in appropriate ways in the appropriate context.

4. The practice of living consciously: To be competent to cope with the basic challenges of life and being worthy of happiness. The experience itself.

5. The practice of living purposely: Identify our short and long term goals and purposes and actions needed to attain them.

6. The practice of personal integrity: Living with congruence between what we know, what we profess, and what we do. Telling the truth, honoring our commitments, exemplifying in action the values we profess to admire.

Goal-Setting:
Look at successful people in their personal and professional lives and you will see goal-setters. Goals are not emotions, yet they certainly can be filled with tremendous emotion. The more passionate you are about a goal, the greater your success will feel when you reach it. I want you to be passionate about losing weight permanently and living a healthy lifestyle. This is a new begin-

ning and this is exciting. Bring that passion to your new goal and your eyes will see the goal in a positive way, and your new attitude will generate new seeds of optimism and enthusiasm.

When we set a goal externally, our inner mind works as a coach to keep us on track with the proper self-talk and expectations. Eventually, the two work as a team to cheer us onto our goal.

Remember Earl Nightengale and his inspiring words: "We become what we thing about most of the time." I want you to think about losing that weight, embarking on a new healthy lifestyle, and with the ingredients liberally laced throughout these pages, you will become that person when you take action. So be specific with the number of pounds you desire to lose and be realistic and enthusiastic.

Here are the six ingredients for your success:
1. Fix in your mind the exact number of pounds you want to lose. For example, you want to lose 30 pounds.

2. Determine exactly what you intend to give in return for the weight loss. For example, you may have to give up your daily two scoops of double double chocolate mocha extra rich and creamy ice cream.

3. Establish a date when you intend to reach your goal. For example, if today is June 1, at a 6 pound loss

per month (a very realistic and healthy weight loss goal and target date) you could be at your target weight by November 1.

4. Create a definite plan for carrying out your goal and begin immediately. For example, write the plan after reviewing the pages you are currently reading.

5. Write out a clear and concise statement of the weight you want to lose and the target date; what you intend to give in return for the weight loss, and describe clearly in detail the plan through which you intend to acquire it. Studies have shown that those people who write out their goals on paper have a 97% chance of reaching their goals.

6. Now you are ready for the fuel that will propel you with enthusiasm. I want you to read your written statement aloud two times daily, once before going to bed at night and once after getting up in the morning. As you read your goal with conviction and optimism and energy, I want you to see and feel and believe yourself as already being that weight, looking and feeling healthy and energetic, and living a healthy lifestyle with power and passion.

CHAPTER 2

▼

FEARS

Today in our society we sometimes look at a "four-letter word" as bad. This can often paralyze us. Take the four-letter word "fail." This one word, put into our subconscious mind, can stop us from taking one step toward the door of life. If the seed of success, which is the opposite of failure, is planted and nourished with the right amount of love, nourishment, sunshine, and other ingredients, then that's what will grow—success. If on the other hand, you plant that pesky, nasty, insidious seed of failure, you don't need any nourishment at all because it will kill all hopes, desires, and dreams without any help. Plant the right seed and the right outcome is out there for you. It is absolutely true and exciting and magical. "Whatever the mind of man can conceive and believe, it can achieve." Leave the belief out of the recipe, and you have nothing. Belief is the yeast that makes the bread, the staff of life, rise. The greater the belief, the greater your potential to reach your goal. Before you can truly believe, you have to understand that pesky seed of failure if you have it deep within your mind, and if so, this understanding can be addressed and the idea of failure can be dismissed.

Let's take a close look at some of these fears. Why do we fear something? If someone asked you if you were afraid to lose weight, you'd probably laugh and initially think that was ridiculous. At closer inspection, it is a wise and insightful question. The answer can lay the groundwork for a solid foundation upon which to begin your new "I believe" mindset; a belief that you can lose the weight you really want to lose, once and for all. Look at failure as a result of an attempt at success. After all, if you don't attempt something, you can't fail, right? Babe Ruth, the greatest baseball player in the game, the true "king of success," was also the "king of failure." If he hadn't swung his bat and missed so many times, he wouldn't have hit the ball successfully so many times. The same strategy and concept applies to Michael Jordan, Tiger Woods, Kobe Bryant and other athletes in their respective sports, and it can apply to you. Change your thinking, keep your eye on the ball of success, your new weight loss goal, and you'll be a winner, a champion, the king or queen of your own game.

Napoleon Hill, in his book "Napolean Hills Keys to Success" believes there are six ghosts of Fear:

- The Fear of Poverty
- The Fear of Criticism
- The Fear of Ill Health
- The Fear of Loss of The Love of Someone
- The Fear of Old Age
- The Fear of Death

Of these six fears, I believe the fear of criticism is the most crucial to losing weight. That's because it destroys initiative and discourages the use of your imagination. It could be the criticism of others, or criticism from the past, or it could be the criticism of the present. The worst form is self-criticism that you let fester within you and paralyze you beyond your control. There's the rub. You really do have control over your internal thoughts, but you are paralyzed in fear. The vibrations of fear from the past pass from one mind to another, the subconscious mind to the conscious mind.

The symptoms of the fear of criticism are:

- Self-Consciousness: Nervousness, timidity, and awkward movements in the hands and body

- Lack of Poise: Lack of voice control and nervousness in the presence of others

- Personality: Lacking in firmness of decision, personal charm and the ability to express opinions of self

- Lack of Initiative: Failure to embrace opportunities for self-advancement and improvement

- Lack of Ambition: Mental and physical laziness and lack of self-assertion

Before you can become successful in your decision to lose weight, your mind must be prepared to receive it. Indecision is the seed of fear. Indecision sprouts into doubt. The two combine together and form fear. Remember this and plant it firmly in your subconscious mind; "fears are nothing more than states of mind." A persons state of mind is subject to control and direction by the owner and controller, and you are the captain, the pilot, and the film director. Man can create nothing which he does not first conceive in the form of an impulse of thought. Mans thought impulses begin immediately to translate themselves into their physical equivalent, whether those thoughts are voluntary or not. Every man and woman has the ability to completely control his own mind and can also shut the door to negative vibrations, utterances, and the words of others. Nature has given man an enormous gift of control and another gift of choice. These two, used simultaneously and in positive and productive endeavors, can be magical and miraculous.

If you accept these gifts, then you can see that fear can be overcome; we can destroy the fear.

Remember that your purpose in life is to achieve successes, small, medium and large; even the new supersize. Your weight loss goal may be small, medium, large, or supersize, the amount is not of paramount importance on day one. What is important, is the fact that you are the master of your own destiny, just as surely as you have the power to control your own thoughts. The choice is yours. Choose wisely.

Here are some strategies to overcome the fear of failure. Ask yourself these three questions about your desire to lose weight permanently.

1. Are your goals, your goals, or are they the goals of others? For example, if you want to lose weight because your spouse wants you to lose weight, you are setting yourself up for failure at the starting gate. The goal must be your goal, for yourself, and it begins by yourself, in the seed of your mind. From there, you can use all the appropriate and applicable ingredients you will be reading about in the Baker's Dozen.

2. Are your goals realistic? If your goal is to lose 50 pounds in 10 weeks, the best word to use here is "unrealistic." If your goal is to lose the 50 pounds by eating with

the same poor habits you now employ, again, "unrealistic." If your goal is to focus only on seeing the pounds melt away without regard to your mind and your spirit, again, "unrealistic."

3. Have you prepared small rewards along your road to weight loss and maintenance? This is important. We learn by repetition and the same strategy can be employed when we reach a mini-goal, such as a five pound weight loss. The rewards of better health, new lifestyle habits, more energy, pride and patience are the best rewards, yet mini goals will help you reinforce your self confidence and they're fun. A good strategy and a super way to reward yourself is to take a number like five, which might match your incremental weight loss goal, and add a $15.00 reward for each 5 pounds lost. That $15.00 is the amount you will spend on the reward. You write each reward on a piece of paper, one for each five pounds lost, put it into a fish bowl and pull one out each time you lose five pounds. Try it. It will make you feel like a kid. A woman might put "buy new nail polish" on one slip of paper and "buy new novel" on another of her papers to toss into her fish bowl. A man might put "buy new kite and go fly the kite" on one slip of paper and "buy one long stemmed red rose for someone special" on another slip of paper for his fish bowl.

Now, take your weight loss goal and do what I call book-ending and begin at the end of the question;

what's the worst case scenario and work your way to the best case scenario. If you've tasted the ingredient of the power of the mind in Chapter I, and you've begun to plant the seeds of success in your subconscious from the beginning of the book up to the present, then you now know that there is no worst case scenario. You can do anything you set your mind to!

Remember this concept about fear; fear is dark, gloomy, and lonely. It makes one hide, retreat from the joys of life, and can harm your spirit of joy. It zaps your energy and enthusiasm. The opposite, love, is love for your self first. Love encourages your adventurous nature, is light, uplifting, and energizing. With an attitude of love, you can create boundless energy, which in turn energizes your spirit to pursue dreams and see things in a light that shines with optimism, determination, and an ocean of creative juices to achieve, not retrieve from life.

Let's take a look at the fear of success. This fear can surely stagnate our spirit and our lives. When we see something in writing, it can help us answer the question in a rational and non-emotional manner. Write out why you fear success. Quite possibly, it could be the fear of the life you'll experience with your new weight loss and new life style habits. This could truly change your life and perhaps this brings on new responsibilities, especially for yourself. Now, change your thoughts and see what happens; you are the most important person in the world and you deserve the best. You cannot help others, those you love with your heart and soul, nor can you help those you touch in a professional manner, if you don't take care of your own needs first. This is not being selfish. This is being smart. Quite frankly, you will be better able to help others when you take care of yourself first. You will have more energy and vitality and this translates into more productivity on your part, not only directed toward yourself, but also toward others.

If that entails new responsibilities, you can handle that too. If you can lose 15 or 20 or 30 pounds, whatever your desired weight loss goal is, you can handle any new responsibilities you may encounter. Remember, your new mindset is one of "I can, because" and "I can, because" holds the seeds of success.

Another possible fear of success relates to guilt. When you're successful with your new lifestyle, you may erroneously feel you don't deserve the success, which is a way to see and feel guilt. You are feeling guilty that you are empowered to be a new you, and that old mindset says you don't deserve success. You should change your attitude to one that says you deserve success in all areas of your life; personally, socially, and professionally. We were given special talents as human beings and each of us has the responsibility to ourselves, to others, and most importantly to the Creator, to reach for the stars, be a shinning star, and never let a success or failure get in our way of living a grand and joyful life.

Napoleon Hill said it well: "Your mind is your Spiritual Estate and protect it with the care to which divine royalty is entitled." You were blessed with willpower. You can control your mind or it can control you. The choice is yours. Choose wisely.

Lloyd Jones said eloquently: "The men who try to do something and fail are infinitely better than those who try nothing and are successful." Dr. Shana Schenker said eloquently: "The men and women who try something today when they failed at that same something yesterday, are truly the successful winners in life."

———— ▼ ————

CHAPTER 3

GOAL-SETTING

Why oh why do we procrastinate? I could give you hundreds of reasons and hundreds of excuses. You want to lose weight and embrace a new lifestyle that will change you internally as well as externally, yet—let's take a look at a few of these bogus excuses.

- I lack willpower
- I've failed so many times before
- What will others say when they see the new me?
- I haven't got the time
- I'm really not that fat
- I've had the fat for so long it's part of me
- I'll do it when the timing is better
- I don't have the support system I need

You can now disregard these and any other excuses you may come up with. With the right seeds in your head, mixed with the right ingredients in the remaining chapters, excuses are just words; words that you made up and should now have no place in your subconscious mind.

Here are five ingredients to propel you to your goal and kick procrastination in the bud permanently. These strategies have been utilized by the most successful people in business. To be successful in any endeavor, we should cash in on the successes of others who have learned from other successful people before them. We don't have to reinvent the wheel here.

1. The night before, make "A To Do List" for your personal life, your professional life, and your weight loss goal.

2. Prioritize. Remember, without your health, mentally and physically, you will lack the energy, drive, and the fuel to set your heart afire toward your new goal, so you should and must be priority #1. If that means that Saturday, tomorrow for example, is gym day, then going to look at a new armoire for the living room is not priority #1.

The next day I want you to post the "To Do List" where you will see it clearly. Now, it's Saturday and you will see that you have a 2 pm gym appointment for your-self. You may also enjoy making a copy for your family, which becomes a reinforcement of your commitment and confidence, and this could become contagious and inspirational for other family members who want to set and achieve their own personal and or professional goals.

3. Divide each goal into sub-goals. This may mean you'll have to stop at the fuel station before the gym and pick up the clothes from the cleaners. No problem, because it's on your "To Do List."

4. Be aware that you're not alone. There are support-ive people all around you and sometimes you should ask for help. Perhaps your teenage daughter has been driving for a few months and she could go to the cleaners for you. This might help her improve her driving skills on a weekend when there's less traffic, and give her a sense of responsibility as well as a good feeling that she can help her mom or dad out.

5. Let's look at persistence, which is a positive word and is actually the opposite of quitting. Remember that "winners never quit and quitters never win." With your new attitude and on your way to being an even bigger success, it shouldn't be difficult to imprint this axiom into your subconscious; "winners never quit and quitters

never win." Be a winner, not a quitter. The feeling is fabulous and the results can be remarkable.

Here are six ingredients to add to your recipe for success.

1. Develop an enthusiastic attitude about yourself and your potential. With the right mindset and other ingredients mixed with enthusiasm, life really will look great even before you've reached your goal, and you'll begin to feel better now.

2. Develop an optimistic attitude that says: "I can do anything I set my mind to." Remember that optimists live longer than pessimists. This is truly food for thought. When you love your new weight and enjoy your new lifestyle, you'll also add more years to your life; now that's a win-win situation!

3. Smile. Sending out a kind word with your smile is like throwing out hugs to people. It's good for others and it's also good for you; now that's a hard combination to beat.

4. Laugh. Laughter really is the best medicine. Remember that laughter is contagious; something that people would really like to catch because it's beneficial to our cardiovascular system and strengthens our health physically and emotionally.

5. Be neotenous. This means be childlike. See life through the eyes of a child. Be curious; be fearless; be flexible; be outrageous; be bold. Dr. Deepak Chopra, in his book "Ageless Body, Timeless Mind," writes; "Being young at heart is a marker of long life." This wisdom is priceless.

6. Get up each day and begin it anew. A new enthusiasm for all the opportunities that are yours to have and to hold. It doesn't cost a thing and yet it is absolutely priceless.

Here's a great story told by Pastor Joel Osteen of The New Lakewood Church in Houston, Texas, on one of his inspirational speeches, which was televised worldwide and touches millions. It aired in April of 2006 and will be timeless in the near and distant future: I call it "The Frog Story:" Two frogs fell into a bowl of milk. The frog on the right kept kicking and kicking and kicking till he thought his legs would wear out. He kept complaining and moaning and groaning and finding every excuse to quit trying to reach the top of the bowl to escape. The frog on the left kept kicking and kicking and kicking till he thought his legs would wear out, yet he looked for every excuse to continue trying. Both frogs became fatigued physically, yet the frog on the right began to fatigue "mentally" as well. Finally, he lost the control, the will, the might to continue, and as he stopped kicking, he fell to the bottom of the bowl. The other frog kept kicking and kicking and kicking and with his mind focused on his goal, he wasn't mentally fatigued at all. Eventually, he felt the milk turn into a different consistency which was thicker, richer, and creamier. Eventually, the liquidy milk turned to cream and the frog jumped out of the bowl.

You're lucky. You have your "Mind-Body-Spirit" Coach here for you and the frogs didn't. Think how high you can go and how far you can jump with a coach on your side.

CHAPTER 4

▼

MOTIVATION

A Tablespoon of motivation is fine, but a full cup is better and will make the journey to your goal more exciting and exhilarating along the way.

The chapter on the mind and the proper attitude is an excellent foundation and an important ingredient for your success. Now, we need a huge cup of motivation. Motivation isn't tangible; it is absolutely intangible and is different for all of us. Motivation comes from within and it's the yeast that makes bread rise; the fuel that pushes you toward your goal.

Let's take a look at the five areas that you must be aware of on a conscious level which will help in the five ingredients that can propel you to a supercharged motivation:

- <u>Thinking</u>
- <u>Habit</u>
- <u>Physiological</u>
- <u>Social</u>
- <u>Emotional Eating</u>

If you are under tremendous stress due to family and or professional commitments, this is a good time to acknowledge how lucky you are to be part of the world of relaxation. In the following chapters, I will elaborate on the different types and their integration into the successful formula. Massage, Deep Relaxation, Diaphramatic Breathing, Meditation, Hypnosis, and Guided Imagery are the top six ingredients.

Remember that your anger, resentment, guilt, or fear are emotions that you can control; these can be detrimental and negative emotions that send you grabbing for unhealthy foods if you live a life of unconscious mindlessness. You can choose the right ingredient, ie. the right relaxation technique, to curb your trigger or triggers and therefore control your hands that reach for the unhealthy foods.

- <u>Thinking</u>: When you think negatively, you put negative toxins into your mind and your thoughts. Thoughts become things. Here, the end result could be more weight on your hips and thighs. An excellent approach is what I call "the stop sign" approach. Whenever you have a negative thought that triggers you to run to the refrigerator or freezer, immediately visualize in your mind a red and white octagonal stop sign. This makes you slow down and stop the negative self talk and negative reaction and negative action. Now, substitute a new and positive thought about yourself. A positive silent affirmation such as, "I love eating healthy foods that give me energy and vibrant health." Repeat this three times and feel the negative thought floating away and the positive thought energizing you to do the right thing; reaching for a juicy red apple instead of a dark detrimental brownie.

- Habit: A habit is a learned response. Some are good and some aren't. Many of the eating habits we engage in are poor. The good news is that a new habit can be established with conscious awareness and an old habit can be extinguished also. A good idea is to keep a log for a few days and write down your eating habits; then you can actually see what needs to be extinguished. The good habits are liberally and deliciously sprinkled throughout these pages. The things you might want to jot down would be; do you eat absentmindedly while watching T.V? Do you eat when you're not really hungry, but boredom sends you to the kitchen prowling for food? Do you clean your large plate, even after you have a feeling of fullness in your stomach? You get the idea.

- Physiological: When we follow a Holistic Approach to health, our physiological needs will be addressed and we won't feel hungry or deprived.

- Social: You may feel pressure due to social situations that tempt you with unhealthy calories. The key ingredient here is choice. You do have a choice as to what you put into your mouth. Armed with the right positive affirmations, visual imagery, and a positive mental attitude about your Holistic Approach to Success, you'll have all the ammunition to say, "No Thank You" in a friendly, yet firm manner. Three words, when spoken graciously and genuinely, can have a positive and powerful effect on your goal to being in control of your health, today and tomorrow. Try it on for size and one day the size of the clothes that you try on will be smaller then the size you are wearing today.

- Emotional: Sometimes when our lives are over- welmed with caring for others personally and possi- bly professionally, the result is treating ourselves unjustly. We then "take care of ourselves" via hand to mouth, with the wrong foods and the wrong amount of the right foods. At other times, when we are overstressed, we reach for a destresser, which could be a donut or cupcake or cookie. It would be far healthier to reach for the right foods, a delicious apple or pear, and a stress reduction technique, which will be found and clarified in an upcoming chapter, which is a win-win for your body and mind and spirit.

Here are five ingredients for a supercharged motivation:

1. <u>Positive Mental Attitude</u>: When we bring a positive mental attitude to the table literally and figuratively, the table of life, we light and ignite our minds and bodies with the proper fuel to go forward to our goal. There are three kinds of fuel at the pumps; unleaded, regular, and premium. Each morning when you rise, I want you to mentally fill your mind with premium fuel; the two P's (Positve and Premium) go together to ignite your motivation.

2. <u>Desire</u>: You must have a burning desire to reach your goal. When you have your health, mentally, physically, and spiritually, you have true wealth. If your desire is to add years to your life, then a burning desire for success, the holistic way, is the best way.

3. <u>Belief</u>: This boils down to what you cause your mind to think and feel certain about, without an ounce

of doubt. If you truly believe that you can achieve a goal, you're already racing toward the finish line of success. This belief must be as firm as a redwood tree and the seed must be planted and nourished in your conscious and subconscious minds.

4. <u>Expectation</u>: When you expect something to happen, you have an inner knowing that you accept with faith. No doubts. No hesitation of thought. No thought is involved because it's a part of your being, just as your right pinky is part of you and your left elbow is part of you. Something that you can see and touch. When we possess this expectancy, we are empowered to create our life with dreams that give us the desire to jump out of bed each morning with a smile on our face because we know it's going to be a great day. We truly can create the life of our dreams, minute by minute, day by day, with the positive energy beginning in our subconscious and then accepted, without doubt, by our conscious, and acted upon, again, without doubt. When we truly expect something to happen, positive or negative, it will. Make yours a positive expectation. You'll be happy you did.

5. <u>Action</u>: Your positive mental attitude is supercharged; you have a burning desire; your belief is unshakable; you expect the best. Now, you need to take your Eighteen Carat Gold Key Card and turn the ignition and go forward. You must take action. There are

three action ingredients that you need in your recipe to put yourself in the right gear to propell yourself toward success.

1.   Plan for Success: Do this the night before. Write down your "Recipe For Success" with the ten most important action items. You now have a clear mind so you can sleep restfully. Also, the act of writing something down has been proven to plant that specific writing in your subconscious just by the very act of taking pencil or pen to paper. It's one of those glorious powers of the mind that helps successful people in their personal and professional lives.

2.   Have your sub-goals and long-term goals posted in your home, car, and office (if applicable) so you will look at them daily and often. This allows you to internalize the good feeling of how you will look and feel when you attain your goal.

3.   Have your Fish Bowl of Rewards clearly displayed in your home so you can see it daily. It's really nice when you know there are small prizes along the way to the big prize. Knowing that in one, two, or three more "lost pounds" you'll "gain" a prize, is fun and neotenous. This is the best of both worlds; creating your success recipe and enjoying it bite by bite

along the way to the new slimmer, trimmer and more energetic you.

CHAPTER 5

▼

STRESS

Stress! Six letters that can affect us physically and psychologically. The reports on stress are truly eye opening. The United States Bonzell Survey found seven out of ten people felt a lot of stress on a typical day and 30% felt tremendous stress. A Gallop Poll found 90% of respondents were stressed at work at least one time a week and 25% on a daily basis. A Prevention Magazine survey found 54% of respondents felt they had more stress in their lives than their parents did. 75% said stress was preventing them from enjoying their lives more.

There are two signs of stress; physical and psychological.

Here are the physical signs of stress:

- Muscle tension and aches
- Tiredness
- Fatigue
- Shakiness
- Lethargy
- Excessive sweating
- Clammy hands
- Dry mouth and throat
- Cold hands and feet
- Frequent urination
- Lowered libido
- Loss of appetite
- Overeating
- Increased use of alcohol, drugs, and or medication
- Nail-biting
- Hair-twirling or hair pulling

Here are the psychological signs of stress:

- Irritability
- Moodiness
- Sadness
- Worry, panic, and feeling upset
- Loss of sense of humor
- Feeling overwhelmed
- Memory lapses
- Difficulties in concentrating
- Feelings of fear
- Difficulties in focusing
- Intrusive and racing thoughts

How can stress make you sick? A 2006 Prevention Magazine article states that 75-90% of all visits to a primary care physician are for complaints and conditions that are in some way stress-related. It also reports that every single week 112 million people take some form of medication for stress-related symptoms. Almost every single bodily function is affected. Your muscles are the primary target of stress. When you are under stress, your muscles contract and they become tense. This muscle tension can affect your nerves, blood vessels, skin, organs, and bones. Muscle spasms, chest pains, and upper and lower back pain can result from stress. It can also play a role in circulatory diseases such as coronary heart disease, sudden cardiac death, and strokes. Stress can increase your blood pressure, constrict your blood vessels, raise your cholesterol level and speed up the rate at which your blood clots. Stress is now considered a major factor in heart disease, right up there with being over-weight, smoking, and lack of exercise.

Heart disease kills more men over the age of 50 and more women over the age of 65 than any other disease. Stress can contribute to GERDS and cause constipation, diarrhea, gas, bloating, and weight loss. Studies have shown that stress affects the immune system.

With this scary news, can stress also be good?

"Stress is the spice of Life," said Hans Selye, a pioneer researcher in the field of stress. He termed the good kind of stress, eustress, as opposed to distress, the bad kind of stress. The eu part of eustress comes from the Greek meaning "good." Stress can be a positive force in your life, like watching a close playoff game, a ride at the amusement park, or falling in love. All of these events can be stressful, yet they can add joy to ones life.

Let's look at a working definition of stress by Albert Ellis, a psychologist, who also established a model of Stress: The ABC Model. "Stress is what you experience when you believe you can't cope effectively with a threatening situation."

A > B > C where:

A is the activating event or stressful situation.

B is the belief, thought, or perception about A.

C is the emotional consequences or stress that results from holding these beliefs.

Let's examine A, B, and C. You can change A. This means modifying your environment. Let's take ants. Stay away from ants. If you work in pest control, then you can change B, the way you perceive them. Much of your stress is self-induced and you can learn to see things differently. What you do is look at the same situation with different eyes, ie. a different perception and a different attitude.

You can change your C. Even if you can't change A and B, you can still manage your stress by mastering other skills. You can learn how to relax your body and quiet your mind. You can learn techniques of becoming calm and actually turn off your stress.

Your point of power is in the present moment. Right here and right now in your mind. It doesn't matter how long you have had a negative thought. The thoughts we've held and the words we've repeatedly used have created our life and experiences up to this point. What we are choosing to think and say today, at this very moment, will create tomorrow, and the next day, week, month and year; the point of power is in the present moment and this is where we begin to makes changes. The smallest beginning will make a big difference.

Picture this scene. You're a baby. You were total love and joy. You felt the world was your oyster. You asked to have your needs met and you openly expressed your emotions of joy, happiness, fear, hurt, hunger, etc. You loved and accepted yourself and every part of your being. You didn't find flaws anywhere. You learned later in life to be influenced in a negative way and the good news is that the negative "stuff" can be unlearned.

To permanently eliminate a condition, we must work to dissolve the mental cause. Before you begin a new positive affirmation, which is the opposite of a negative affirmation, you need to work on your willingness to release the need for excess weight, for example. When the need is gone, the outer effect must die. No plant can live if the root is cut away.

The negative mental thought patterns that cause most disruptions in the mind are self-criticism, anger, guilt, and resentment. Look at self-criticism. If you are consistently criticizing yourself in having no control over your eating habits, this can lead to low self-esteem and anger turned inward. On the inside, you'll punish yourself with negative self-talk and on the outside you'll punish yourself by grabbing for another donut or cookie because you don't believe you deserve to have a slim body. The guilt seeks punishment and you continue to punish yourself with poor food choices and poor lifestyle habits.

The two keys to stopping the vicious cycle are to:

- Find your trigger (for example, I eat because I come from a large family and they won't love me if I don't finish all the food on my plate)

- Look inside yourself to whether you have self-criticism, anger, resentment, or guilt

Now, acknowledge them openly and allow your subconscious mind to work with you to create a new you. Write positive affirmations with belief and conviction and say them aloud five to ten times daily. Look in the mirror, into your eyes, and say them with passion, energy, and belief. This is your mental workout. Here are three positive affirmations for you to chew on now.

> "I feel slim and trim."
> "A teaspoon of optimism makes me catapult to success."
> "I choose to eat healthy foods daily."

Here is a dynamic quote from Paramahansa Yogananda: "So long as we believe in our heart of hearts that our capacity is limited and we grow anxious and unhappy, we are lacking in faith. One who truly trusts in G-D has no right to be anxious about anything."

If you want to experience the second half of this quote, you truly can live a tranquil and stress-free life. When you're in a mental state of joy, you're at peace with all things. In this state of joy, you feel fulfilled in all facets of your life.

Being stressed is not a natural state of being. You have the inner power to create a stress-free life. You can utilize this power to attract, like a magnet, joy or frustration, peace or anxiety. There is no actual stress in the outer environment; only in your inner mental environment. It's your thoughts that create this concept of stress. Stress isn't something that you can package and sell. You can't touch it or smell it. There are, however, millions of people who choose to engage in negative thinking. When we think stressfully, we create reactions in the body to grab our attention. The signals may be nausea, stomach tension, headaches, ulcers, elevated blood pressure, increased heart rate and hundreds of other feelings, from a minor discomfort to a serious life-threatening illness. We speak as if stress is in the outside world with the ability to attack us. Yet, stress in our body is the result of our reaction to a situation and our negative choice of how to deal with the situation. Remember, you have free choice. You can accept a thought as stressful or not. It's a habit; a good habit if you choose to think positive thoughts and a bad habit if you choose to think negative thoughts.

Here's a positive thought! The next time you find yourself in a potentially stressful situation, such as a holiday dinner where the pressure to overeat unhealthy foods seems overwhelming, say these five magic words: "I choose to feel good." Say them silently and then out-loud. By saying these five words, you receive two benefits. Firstly, you'll begin to feel tranquil and stress-free. Secondly, in this positive state, you will make the proper food choices and feel better physically, as well as mentally. You can take five magic words, and with practice and a new habit, change your thinking and change your life.

Eight ingredients for living a stress-free life:
1. Remember that your natural state is one of joy. You are a product of love and joy.

2. Your thoughts, not the Universe, cause your stress. Your thoughts activate stressful reactions in your body. Stressful thoughts create resistance to joy and happiness. These thoughts include: "I can't." "I'm afraid." "I'm too fat." "I don't deserve it." etc. These destructive thoughts are like a mental program to resist a state of tranquility and peace.

3. You can change your thoughts of stress in any given moment and eliminate the stress for the next few minutes or hours or days. By making a conscious decision to distract yourself from worry, you've begun the process of stress-reduction.

4. Monitor your stressful thoughts by checking on your emotional state right in the moment. Ask yourself: "Do I feel good right now?" If the answer is in the negative, repeat your five magic words: "I choose to feel good." Say them with conviction; say them with energy; say them with belief; say them with pride; say them with passion.

5. Choose a thought that will activate good feelings. Ask yourself if the thought feels good. If not, choose one that does feel good. Consider this thought: "I'm too fat." Now, eliminate that thought and substitute "I'm slim." Remember the fact that "thoughts become things."

6. Spend time observing babies and emulate their joy. They love everyone. They have no resistance to being filled with total joy. They don't need a reason to be happy. Try it and you might be amazed at the incredible feelings that will rush over you; feelings of sheer, pure, beautiful joy.

7. Practice being in silence and meditation. Nothing relieves stress and anxiety and all forms of negative low energy emotions like silence and meditation. This positive habit practiced once or twice a day can literally add years to your life and life to your years. An exhaustive study was conducted in the 1970's involving hundreds

of adults from different backgrounds and cultures and the conclusions were incredible. Those from the medical and holistic worlds combined their expertise and concluded that people who engage in meditation for a minimum of twenty minutes daily for five years can decrease their biological age by twelve years. Yes, this is amazing and it is true. Be true to yourself and begin meditating so you can improve the quality of your life and possibly expand your horizons in other areas of your life.

8. Stay in a state of gratitude and awe. You can't feel appreciative and stressed at the same time because these are two opposite emotions. Our subconscious will only accept one at a time, so choose wisely. "You should feel good not because the world is right, but your world should be right because you feel good." Powerful words from Dr. Wayne Dyer.

CHAPTER 6

▼

RELAXATION TECHNIQUES

Buddha was so wise. "A journey of one thousand miles begins with the first step."

The first step may be the hardest, yet it can propel you to experiences that can change your life. Let's take a look at three ingredients that can evaporate your stress into the Universe.

    1   A = awareness of the stress. Know what your stress looks like and where it comes from.

    2   A = analysis of the stress. Determine the best way to manage the stress.

3   A = action. You have to move toward the stress to eliminate it and that is what this chapter will address.

Techniques and Tools to reduce your stress.

Progressive Relaxation:
The following technique is highly effective and has been proven to be a valuable tool for quickly reducing muscle tension and promoting relaxation.

(1) Lie down or sit as comfortably as you can and close your eyes. Find a quiet, dimly lit location that gives you some privacy for a while.

(2) Tense the muscles of a particular body part. Begin by simply making a fist. As you clench your fist, notice the tension and strain in your hand and forearm. Without releasing that tension, bend your right arm and flex your biceps, making a muscle as if you were a kid on the playground and wanted to impress a friend. Do not strain yourself in any of these muscle tensing exercises; do not over do it. When you tense a muscle group, tense about three-quarters of what you can actually do. If you feel pain or soreness, ease up on the tension or delay your practice for another time.

(3) Hold the tension in the body part for about seven seconds.

(4) Let go of the tension, fairly quickly, letting the muscles go limp.
Notice the difference in the way your hand and arm feels. Notice the difference in feelings between the sensations of tension and those of relaxation. Let those feelings of relaxation deepen for about thirty seconds.

(5) Repeat steps #1 through #4, substituting a different muscle group each time. Continue with your left hand and arm and then work your way through another major muscle group.

Autogenic Training:
Two other synonyms for autogenic training would be "self generation" and "mind over body." Autogenic training attempts to regulate your autonomic nervous system (your heart rate, blood pressure, and breathing, among other things) rather than relaxing your muscles. You use your mind to regulate your bodies internal stress levels. It is truly an amazing concept and what is even more amazing is the fact that it actually works. Monks have been demonstrating the awesome power of the mind for years. They immerse their bodies into a pool of icy cold water. They then train their minds to create perspiration inward and this internal heat dries the cold wet

moisture on the outside of their bodies; it is hard to believe, unless you choose to believe, and then and only then can you create amazing changes in your life using your mind the way the monks do, substituting your particular goals, not those of the monks.

Autogenic Training relies on the power of suggestion to induce a physiological change within you. These suggestions are mental images that your subconscious mind picks up and transmits to your body. Just thinking about certain changes in your body produces those kinds of changes. As an end result, you are able to experience deep feelings of relaxation.

Here are the ingredients and a recipe for Autogenic Training. It takes about 30 minutes, worth every second invested in your time. Get comfortable. Find a quiet place. Sit or lie down, yet support your body. Breathe slowly and smoothly and begin to feel a calm within your body. Concentrate passively. Be aware of your body and mind, but don't analyze anything. Should a distracting thought come your way, notice it and let it go. Allow various body parts to begin feeling warm and heavy. Begin by focusing on your right arm and say slowly and softly to yourself the following words:

"I am calm ... I am at peace ... my right arm is warm ... and heavy ... I can feel the warmth and heaviness flowing into my right arm ... I can feel my right arm becoming warmer and heavier ... I can feel my right arm becoming warmer and heavier ... I am at peace ... I am calm ... I am at peace ... I am calm." Take time to become aware of the feelings in your arm and hand. Notice that your right arm is actually becoming warmer and heavier. After you repeat the above phrases, remain silent and calm for a minimum of thirty seconds. Then, focus your attention on your left arm. Repeat the same phrases again, but this time you will substitute your left arm for your right arm. Move to the other parts of your body, using the same words for each body part. The sequence is as follows: Right arm, left arm, then both arms. Right leg, left leg, then both legs. Neck and shoulders, then your chest and abdomen. Finally, your entire body. The whole sequence should take approximately 30 minutes, but feel comfortable with extending your relaxation experience for another 15 or 30 minutes if you have the time and desire to do so. It's like being on a mini vacation, without the hassle of going to the airport or train station or making reservations at the closest spa. You have all the ingredients before you so enjoy and relax.

Here are five mini recipes of relaxation that can be done in half the time, yet are still very effective.

"Heat me Up"
Imagine that the body part you want to focus on,

your arm or left shoulder, is wrapped in a heating pad. Slowly but surely the heat permeates your body, relaxing your muscles more and more.

"Get in Hot Water"

Imagine that you are immersing a body part you want to relax, such as your right ankle or left hand, in very soothing warm water.

"Sunnyside Up"

Mentally direct a sunlamp to a particular part of your body, such as as your right arm or your chest area.

"Heavy Metal"

Visualize weights attached to a particular body part, such as your right leg or your left shoulder.

"Get the Lead In"

Imagine that your body part, your right arm or your left leg, is filled with lead.

Massage

For thousands of years, some form of massage or "laying on of hands," has been used to heal and soothe the sick. To the Ancient Greek and Roman Physicians, massage was one of the principle means of relieving pain. In the 5th Century B.C., Hippocrates, the "Father of Medicine" wrote: "The physician must be experienced in many things, but assuredly, in rubbing. For rubbing can bind a joint that is too loose and loosen a joint that is too rigid."

Relaxation is a transformation of your energy. Normally, your energy is motivated and moving toward a goal. Yet, there is another side to energy, unmotivated energy. The goal is in the present versus long-term motivated goals. When the goal is not in the future, there is nothing to be achieved. This moment is relaxation. Relaxation can start with the body and move to the mind.

Here are six Relaxation recipes to whip up and enjoy. Except for Self-Message and Aromatherapy, which you can do on your own, I strongly recommend that you see a trained professional for the remaining four Massages.

Self-Massage, Head Massage, Reiki, Shiatsu, Chinese Massage, and Aromatherapy.

Self-Massage.

You can massage your hands, feet, face, shoulders, and any other part of your body that needs relaxing. It is a good idea to use oils and warm them to room temperature. (See Aromatherapy for an explanation of the benefits of oils).

Lower the lights to create a relaxing atmosphere.

Apply pressure lightly, then increase slightly. Finish up with lighter pressure.

Linger for a while after the massage to extend the benefits of the relaxation.

Head Massage

This massage tones the muscles and releases tension and stress from the head down throughout your body. Tension in the muscles is released, dispersing toxins, reducing mental and physical stress, and improving blood flow to the brain.

This massage takes approximately 30 to 40 minutes, yet can be extended to 45 or 60 minutes if you prefer.

Reiki

Reiki Massage relaxes you by opening up emotional blocks and you come into closer contact with suppressed feelings and often negative emotions as well. They are energies which can transform themselves into creative forces as soon as you own them and give them attention and expression.

This massage should be given by a trained professional and a full treatment will last from 60 to 90 minutes.

Shiatsu

This massage allows the self to respond naturally to any sensations or emotions that may arise and consciously "let go" into the experience. Few words are spoken during the massage by either person in the room.

This massage should be given by a trained professional. The treatment will last from 30 to 40 minutes.

Chinese Massage

This type of Oriental Massage uses manipulation on specific accupressure points and channels to remove Qi-blood stagnation. The Oriental Medical Treatments, going back thousands of years, focus on twelve channels in a person's body, different channels leading to different body parts. To illustrate, one channel will address the liver while another channel will address the stomach, and so on. They believe that when a channel is blocked, illness results because the blood is prevented from flowing through the body and bringing vital nutrients to nourish and heal the body. The goal of the massage is to open the channels and balance the yin and yang energies, thus promoting good health and well being. There are twelve channels and the goal is to bring the body into balance by opening the channels and letting the blood flow freely while creating balance and harmony for good health.

A trained professional is the key here and the time for a treatment can be 60 to 90 minutes.

Aromatherapy.

You have the ability to massage your stress away with oils. Think of the concept of mind over matter. Your bodies various responses to stress are lined to the hypothalamus in your brain. This part of your brain controls many functions in your body. Since the hypothalamus is part of your limbic system which produces smell, Aromatherapy goes directly to ease your stress.

Relaxing fragrances, the ones that help you deal better with stress, tend to produce slower frequency brain waves (Delta Waves) and they also prompt some Theta Waves. Both Delta and Theta Waves bring out your quiet meditative side. Many of these relaxing aromas also increase another type of brain wave, the Alpha Waves.

According to CNV testing, the aromas of lavender, bergamot, marjoram, sandalwood, lemon, chamomile, and valerian, in that order, produce sedating brain patterns in your brain.

Here are seven advantages of using Aromatherapy:

- To stimulate the immune system
- To reduce stress
- To relax you
- To utilize a technique that works quickly
- To utilize a technique that is inexpensive

- To utilize a technique that works with you, not against you

- To utilize a technique that has few side effects, all of them positive

Enjoy and relax with the following three minute recipes. Although each recipe only takes three minutes to mix the magic potion, the relaxing effect, after application, could last for three hours.

"Relax Away"
    1 drop Chamomile Oil
    5 drops Lavender Oil
    1 drop Ylang Ylang Oil
    Combine for 3 minutes and apply to temples, wrists, elbows, or any areas that appeal to you.

"Meditation and Inner Focus"
    8 drops Sandalwood Oil
    1 drop Rose Oil
    Combine for 3 minutes and apply to temples, wrists, elbows, or any areas that appeal to you.

A Breath of fresh air.

When you came into the world, you came in breathing. Breathing is the most important activity that you do. You can live for days without water and weeks without food, but only a few moments without breathing. Breath is your most powerful friend—your best friend.

The Sanskrit word for "Life Force," prana, is synonymous with the word "breath."

Proper breathing can relax you and revitalize you.

Because breathing affects your state of mind, you can utilize breathing techniques to cultivate a different state of mind. You can change the mood you are in by "conscious breathing." It is also referred to as "Breath Awareness."

Your brain requires more oxygen than most other parts of your body.

Supply it with the oxygen it needs to get more clarity of thought and have longer periods of concentration. Better breathing also affects your overall sense of well being. You feel happier, more alive, and more vibrant.

Here are five benefits of "Conscious-Mindful Breathing," which is also referred to as "Yoga Breathing."

Oxygenation:

One of the greatest benefits of Yoga Breathing is the oxygenation of all the cells in your body. The supply of oxygen to your brain and the muscles of your body increases. Oxygen travels the bloodstream by attaching to the hemoglobin in the red blood cells. This oxygen enables your body to metabolize vitamins, minerals, and other vital nutrients your body needs.

Detoxification:

Your lungs are critical to daily detoxification. When you exhale, you release carbon dioxide that has been passed from your bloodstream into your lungs. Carbon dioxide is a waste product of your bodies natural metabolism. By expelling air from the deepest recesses of your lungs, you expel more carbon dioxide and you enable your lungs to take in more oxygen.

Organ Massage:

Each time you inhale, your diaphragm expands. This action massages your heart, intestine, and other organs near your diaphragm. Proper breathing helps to promote improved circulation in these organs.

Posture:

The breathing techniques encourage good posture. Poor posture can be a cause of incorrect breathing. It also strengthens and tones your abdominal muscles.

Metabolism:

Breathing well is supportive to the function of the digestive, respiratory, circulatory, and hormonal systems. Yoga Breathing may be helpful in promoting your metabolic balance in everyday living and keep your body weight in check.

According to Yoga tradition, each person is allotted a certain number of breaths, and after you exceed your number, your time on earth is completed. People who breathe hurriedly and shallowly use up their allotment of breaths quickly, yet if you breath consciously and slowly, your breath allotment lasts for many years. By breathing properly, you have the opportunity to add more years to your life.

Developing a balanced, steady, rhythmic breath, one that is deep and full, helps you live a longer life. Now that's a recipe for life!

The breath is the bridge between the mind and the body. You can do these exercises while sitting, standing, or lying down. I encourage you to have fun and experiment with a variety of exercises. Choose the one you enjoy the most or try different exercises on different days of the week. The exact recipe is up to you. You can be the creative cook in your own kitchen of healthy lifestyle habits.

Seven Guidelines for Happy Breathing:

- Breathe through your nose, unless I instruct you otherwise

- Listen to yourself breath

- Breathe rhythmically

- Concentrate on making a smooth transition between each inhalation and exhalation

- Never force your breath beyond the natural capacity of your lungs

- Don't practice Yoga Breathing in uncomfortable places where the air is too hot or too cold

- Maintain straight posture

Seven different Recipes for Yoga Breathing:

The Complete Breath:

This is a great way to relieve stress and tension. It improves the quality and quantity of the oxygen that enters your body. It is the basis of all breathing techniques. Ideally, you should inhale and exhale six times per minute when using the Complete Breath. Breathing through your nostrils, you inhale 4 to 6 counts at a minimum and you exhale 6 to 10 counts at a minimum.

Three Steps to The Complete Breath:
(1) While sitting, lying down, or standing, relax your shoulders and look straight ahead or close your eyes.

(2) Inhaling slowly through your nose, feel your abdomen and your upper chest gently expand until you fill your lungs to capacity.

(3) Exhaling slowly through your nose, gently engage your abdomen. Practice the Complete Breath ten times, inhaling to a count of 4 and exhaling to a count of 6.

The Abdominal Breath:
Do the Abdominal Breath when you are feeling stress, tension, or fatigue. The relaxing feeling is great.

Five Steps to The Abdominal Breath:
(1) Sit comfortably in a chair or lie on your back.

(2) Place one hand on your abdomen just above your pubic bone and below your navel. Place the other hand on your solar plexus right beneath your breastbone.

(3) Listening to your breath, inhale slowly and deeply through your nostrils, so deeply that your belly expands and you feel a wave of breath moving into the bottom of your lungs.

(4) At the bottom of your inhalation, find the point of transition where your inhale becomes your exhale.

(5) To a count of 6 to 8 seconds, exhale fully through your nostrils.

Feel your entire body relaxing and releasing tension.

Do 10 slow abdominal breaths. Because of the intensity of the relaxation response, do not attempt this technique while driving a car.

The Ocean Breath, also known as "Rib Breathing"
The Ocean Breath oxygenates your blood. It stimulates your circulation and gives you a burst of energy. You emit a sound during the Ocean Breath, the sound of the ocean, its namesake.

Five Steps to the Ocean Breath.
(1) Sit or stand comfortably with your spine straight.

(2) Place your arms on your chest with the fingers of your right hand tucked into your left armpit and the fingers of your left hand tucked into your right armpit.

(3) Close your eyes or look straight ahead with your windpipe open, your jaw and mouth relaxed, and your chin pointing gently downward.

(4) Inhale to a count of 6 to 10, engaging the muscles in the back of your throat as if you are sipping through a straw and feel your ribs open and your breath filling to the top of your lungs.

(5) Gently exhale steadily through your nostrils until the exhale is complete.

Take 10 Ocean Breaths ... Pause to rest ... Do 10 more ... pause.

Do 10 more for a total of 30 breaths.

Balancing Breath:
This is a good relaxation technique to use when you are tired.

Three Steps to The Balancing Breath:
(1) Sit, lie down, or stand with your shoulders, mouth, and jaw relaxed. Close your eyes. Look ahead. Your back should be straight, but not stiff.

(2) To a count of four, slowly inhale through your nose.

(3) To a count of four, slowly exhale through your nose drawing your abdomen gently in and up to help send the breath slowly out. Practice 6 to 10 times, inhaling to a count of 4 and exhaling to a count of 4 ... pause for a count of 10. Then, do another 6 to 10.

Alternate Nostril Breath:
This is an exciting Yoga Breath because the benefits are wonderful. The Alternate Nostril Breath offers physical and subtle effects. Each breath is associated with one cerebral brain hemisphere. The right nostril is associated with the right brain hemisphere where your spatial perceptions begin and the left nos-

tril is associated with the left brain hemisphere where verbal skills are. In traditional Yoga, the right nostril is considered the warming and energetic one and the left nostril is considered the cooling and calming one.

Practice Alternate Nostril Breath to calm your mind and nervous system in times of stress. It induces a powerful sense of well-being in the present moment and increases your mental clarity and alertness.

Here are the Four Steps:

(1) Sit comfortably with your eyes closed.

(2) Close your right nostril by pressing your nose gently with your right thumb and then inhale through your left nostril to a count of 4.

(3) Close your left nostril by gently pressing with your right pinky finger and ring finger into your nose. At the same time, remove your thumb from your right nostril and exhale through your right nostril to a count of 8.

(4) Repeat the breath, but this time close your left nostril and inhale through your right to a count of 4, then close your right nostril and exhale to a count of 8 through your left nostril. Start by doing 6 to 10 complete Alternate Nostril Breaths. It requires five to eight minutes of concentrated breathing.

Cleansing Breath:

The purpose of this Yoga technique is to cleanse out your lungs and therefore, the best place and time to perform it is in the morning in the fresh dewy air.

The Two Steps to The Cleansing Breath:
(1) Inhale a complete breath comfortably through your nostrils to a count of 4 to 6.

(2) Gently purse your lips as you strongly exhale to a count of 4.

Exhale vigorously as you make a loud "whoosing" sound. Complete the Cleansing Breath 4 to 6 times.

This is the most dynamic of the Yoga Breaths. It sends energy to all parts of your body and you feel more vibrant and alive.

Here are The Four Steps:
(1) Stand upright with your feet spread wider than your hips and toes, toes pointed forward.

(2) While inhaling a complete breath through your nostrils to a count of 4, extend your arms straight out in front of you with your palms facing upward.

(3) Exhale slowly through your mouth or through your pursed lips as you draw your hands through your

body along the sides of your ribcage and gradually contract the muscles of your arms and hands.

(4) Relax your arms and hands as you inhale deeply. Slowly unclench your fists and return to your starting position.

Repeat steps #2 through #4 six to eight times. Complete 6 to 8 times.

The Body-Mind Connection. It is powerful and magical. You have the incredible ability to exercise your body and mind simultaneously. You can calm the mind so you can receive the full benefits of your mind working with your body in a synergistic way utilizing a strategy that hypnotherapists and others in the healing arts have been practicing for years.

The strategy is called Visualization, sometimes referred to as Guided Imagery.

Visualization occurs when you go on a mental journey with your eyes closed as a means of calming your thinking and achieving a quiet meditative state of self-awareness. You become the writer, director, and producer of your own mental movies. The purpose is to reach a state of deep relaxation and focus. You will need a minimum of 15 minutes to receive the wonderful benefits of visualization, yet 30 minutes is like going to your favorite movie and seeing it twice. Try it for 15 minutes and I guarantee you that you will want to see the second show-ing.

The Ten Ingredients of Visualization:
(1) Lie down or sit comfortably in a chair. Find a quiet and peaceful place for you mental movies.

(2) Notice the tip of your nose and the coolness or warmth of each breath as the stream of air flows in and out of your nostrils.

(3) Keeping the attention on the tip of your nose, feel the sensations of your lungs as they fill with air and then empty themselves with air. Focus on your lungs for at least six breaths.

(4) Imagine that the innermost center of your body, from your hips up to your shoulders, is a deep pond.

(5) View this pond in your mind and direct your attention to the surface of the pond.

(6) Notice the currents or waves in the surface of the pond and look toward the sky, above the pond in your mind, and observe any clouds.

(7) Visualize dropping a pebble into the pond. Follow the pebble as it sinks into the pond.

(8) As the pebble continues to sink, feel a sense of your own depth, the calmness within you and the stilling and quieting of your mind as the pebble falls into deeper waters of inner knowing.

(9) Imagine the pebble coming to rest on the bottom of the pond. Dwell here for as long as you wish.

(10) In the role of the observer, step back from this visualization and notice that you have taken your thoughts into deeper waters.

Dwell comfortably and securely in this place of calm for as long *as* you want to. Remember, you can visit here anytime you want to relax. Visit often and make the visit a grand journey in your life.

CHAPTER 7

▼

HYPNOSIS

Hypnotherapy:

Because of my profession as a Doctor of Clinical Hypnotherapy, as well as having certifications as a Medical Hypnotherapist (C.M.H.), a Hypno-Anesthesia Therapist (Ct.H.A.), and a Hypnotic Anaesthesiologist (H.A.), along with certifications in Weight Loss and Management, Sports Improvement, and Smoking Cessation, I am most passionate about the incredibe benefits of Hypnosis. I speak with passion in my heart, and from experience with my patients, when I say that Hypnosis is a "Miracle of the Mind." There is nothing else like it on Earth or the other Planets in the Solar System. It is more dynamic than a computer and will go with you whereever you go, without batteries, wires, or special carrying cases. Read this chapter over and over again, and you will be enligtened, enthralled, and empowered to change your attitude and change your life when you understand the power of the mind. Read this chapter of Ingredients. Digest the Ingredients. Swallow the Ingredients. You will feel and see some remarkable changes in your life. Enjoy and savor eat and every bite.

People are fascinated with the possibilities of Hypnosis and I would like to give you some history and background on this incredible field I am so proud to be a part of. Thousands of studies have been conducted going back hundreds of years, yet I will only touch on a few key points so you will see the efficacy of this field, which has had its share of bad press and narrow-minded non-medical implications and accusations.

The origins of Hypnotherapy date back to the healing practices of ancient Greece and Egypt. Many religions, such as Judaism, Christianity, Islam, and others, have attributed trance-like behavior to spiritual or divine possession.

Franz Mesmer (1734-1815) was an Austrian physician who is regarded as being the first person to investigate the idea of hypnotherapy in the realm of the world of science to treat many health conditions. He received his medical degree from the Univeristy of Vienna in 1766 and in 1779 he began to treat a variety of health conditions using hypnotherapy. His techniques became the foundation for modern-day hypnotherapy.

Mesmer's technique appeared to be quite successful in the treatment of his patients, but because his personality was seemingly eccentric, the medical profession looked at him with ridicule and scorn. A commission was formed to investigate Mesmer and the panel included the distinguished American Benjamin Franklin and the French physician Jacques Guillotin. Although the commission acknowledged that patients "did appear to obtain noticeable relief from their conditions," the whole idea was dismissed as being nothing more than medical quackery.

It took more than two hundred years for hypnotherapy to become incorporated into medical treatment. The British Medical Association (BMA) approved the use of hypnotherapy as a valid and "orthodox" medical treatment in 1955 and the American Medical Association (AMA) gave its approval three years later in 1958.

The purposes for hypnotherapy are varied and exciting. It is used in a number of fields, including surgery, dentistry, research, psychotherapy, and medicine. Hypnotherapy is commonly used as an alternative treatment for a wide range of health conditions, including, but not limited to, weight loss and control, smoking cessation, and pain management. It is also used to control pain in such conditions as arthritis, headache, childbirth, burns, musculoskeletal disorders, and many more. Hypnotherapy is being used to replace anesthesia, particularly for patients who are allergic to anesthetic drugs, for surgeries such as cesarean sections, hysterectomies, certain cardio-vascular procedures, and others. In the field of dentistry, hypnotherapy has been successfully used on patients who are allergic to all types of novocaine drugs. People who are under stress, those who suffer from anxiety and worry, those who are depressed, those who suffer from sexual performance anxiety, and people who lack self confidence, have all been successfully helped by hypno-therapy. The areas in ones personal and professional life that can be enhanced and helped with hypnotherapy are extensive and nothing short of fantastic.

Hypnotherapy is also used for nonmedical patients who have a desire to overcome bad habits such as nail biting and procrastination. Hypnotherapy has been suc-cessful for people who suffer from performance anxiety on the personal level and in the professional level in areas such as sports and speaking in public. In the academic realm, it has been used successfully to help with learning, classroom participation, improving memory and con-centration, studying, and passing exams such as The BAR EXAM, The CPA EXAM, The Real Estate Brokers Exam, The Pilots Exam, and The Civil Service Exam, to name several of many state licensing exams.

Simply put, Hypnotherapy can be described as achiev-ing a psychological state of awareness that is different from the ordinary state of consciousness. This state of consciousness can be achieved by relaxing the body, focusing on one's breathing, and shifting attention away from the external environment. In this state, the patient has a heightened receptivity to suggestion. The usual procedure for inducing a hypnotic trance in another person is by direct command repeated in a soothing and monotonous tone of voice.

The following five conditions should be present to successfully achieve a state of hypnosis:

- willingness to be hypnotized

- rapport between the patient and the hypnotherapist

- belief on the part of the patient

- motivation on the part of the patient

- a comfortable environment conducive to relaxation

Hypnosis is one of the most potent of ingredients in the holistic approach to permanent weight-loss and a healthy lifestyle. With an open mind and an attitude that is positive and filled with belief, you can transform your current position of excess weight physically and mentally, to a newer, vibrant, slimmer, and healthier you. It all begins in the mind; your mind. As your "Mind-Body-Spitit" Coach, I profess with my heart and soul, try it. Not only will you have the opportunity to lose the "old baggage" once and for all, you will also have an opportunity to see and feel things in a new light. You can lift your spirits, energize your body, and become a true gold medal winner in the winner's circle.

The gateway to this new lifestyle that beckons you is relaxation, and the golden key that opens the gate is hypnosis.

There are several important components to address before a successful session can begin. A person can see a certified hypnotherapist initially and then learn how to induce self-hypnosis. Because self-awareness is important, I want you to read on.

First and foremost, what is your motivation for losing weight? There are basically four areas to explore.

1. To feel better

2. To look better

3. For health considerations

4. To stop allowing food to control you

The key word to truly focus on is "you." Remember that the stronger "your" motivation and the stronger "your" belief that you can succeed, the more receptive your mind will be; if you believe it and conceive it in your mind, you can achieve it.

The next area to address is your learning style. People learn primarily by one of three systems. These systems are auditory, visual, and touch (kinesthetic). We predominate in one of the three, yet we can and often do roll over some of the other two systems into our core system of learning. If you are an auditory, you will learn best by hearing and listening. If you are visual, you will learn best by seeing and reading. If you are kinesthetic, you will learn best by doing and touching. The system analysis will be used in Guided Imagery and Suggestive Therapy to help you train your subconscious mind in the way it prefers to receive information.

The final area to become aware of are the cues that "trigger" your hands to put unneeded and unhealthy food in your mouth.

There are Five Specific Triggers.

1.   <u>Social</u>:

Man is a social being and this is good, unless the pressure is detrimental to one's health. Sometimes other people urge you to eat and you give in to their needs for an eating companion at the ice cream parlor or to make other people at a party feel good that you are joining in at the buffet table.

2.   <u>Situational</u>:

Sometimes you'll pass by a pizza stand and the enticement is too strong for you to pass up. The next thing you know, you're having a pizza with all the toppings of the day and your hips and waistline will show it tomorrow.

3. <u>Physiological</u>:
You may feel hungry even though you recently ate a very full and plentiful meal.

4. <u>Thinking</u>:
It is common to make 101 excuses why you'll eat that cookie or brownie now and start your diet tomorrow, or a week from this weekend, or some day and date in the future.

5. <u>Emotional</u>:
Any emotion, good or bad, can send you to the refrigerator or fast food place; a happy feeling, a sad feeling, an anxious feeling.

Some self insight is necessary here. A Certified Hypnotherapist is a good place to start, because you will be given a series of assessment tests and the results will show, among other things, your learning style and your triggers. If you prefer to use your own initiative, I suggest the following: Sit down in a quiet place without any interruptions or distractions. With pen and paper, begin a "Food Trigger Journal." Create 14 days (a page or two for each of the 14 days) for your daily meals. On the top of the page, put a scale of 1 to 10, 1 standing for "not intense" and 10 standing for "very intense." This will symplify your writing. Now, for the next 14 days, I want you to concentrate not on the the exact foods that you ate at each meal, rather what triggered you into the world of overeating and unhealthy eating. For example, if you had an argument with a family member and that sent you to the freezer looking for the ice cream carton and you proceeded to eat 2 or 3 scoops of ice cream, write this down. Give it a number and come back to this chapter and you will see that this is an "emotional trigger." If you are at a party and your relatives urge you to have seconds as well as two different desserts, and you were really content with one portion and actually not hungry for the desserts, this is referred to as a "situational trigger." When you read through your notes, you'll get the idea. Now, after 14 days of consciously focusing on your habits, you will see a pattern. You might be a situational and emotional eater. You might be a thinking eater and this has allowed you to think your way to a weight that you are ashamed of. The purpose of this exercise is to make you aware of your trigger or triggers and help you design your Guided Imagery and Direct Suggestions to address your own particular needs. If you decide to see a Certified Hypnotherapist, please ask if he or she will be giving you a series of "Self Assessment Tests." If the answer is no," say "thank you" and keep looking until you find one who does. I am constantly told by my patients that they went to a "group weight loss program" for one session because it was inexpensive. They were terribly upset because it didn't work. In hypnosis, you get what you pay for. The main reasons group does not work is because the "hypnotist" is not addressing your individual triggers and learning style. The key word here is "hypnotist" and your goal should be creating an opportunity to become involved with a "hypnotherapist." The other reason these group sessions don't work is because hypnosis is not a one stop fixit experience. When the right ingredients for the individual are addressed, hypnosis works! (A personalized program based on a series of assessment tests; several sessions with the hypnotherapist; reinforcement between sessions by the patient after he or she has been taught how to self-hypnotize; positive rapport between the hypnotherapist and the patient, are all key ingredients to create a great recipe for success in the wonderful world of hypnotherapy.)

There are five things I want you to know about Hypnosis.

- You are not asleep
- You are not unconscious
- You will not lose control
- You won't do anything you don't want to do
- It works

What is Hypnosis?

Hypnosis is a deeply focused state that makes you more acutely aware of suggestions and allows you to be more receptive to those suggestions. For Hypnosis to be effective, try to adopt an open, non-critical attitude. Don't fight the process. It can be a wonderful experience for you and I want you to enjoy it.

Here are Thirteen (a Baker's Dozen) examples of Direct Suggestions:

"I love eating small portions of food"

"I feel energized when I eat healthy foods"

"I love eating slowly and savoring each bite of food"

"I control what goes into my mouth"

"I only eat enough food to satisfy my small appetite"

"I savior eat bite and eat slowly"

"I put my eating utensils down between every bite"

"I enjoy eating to live, not living to eat"

"I am empowered to control my destiny; a slimmer, trimmer, healthier me"

"I feel slim, trim, and vibrantly energized"

"I feel terrific"

"I chew each bite several times before swallowing"

"I feel free and fabulous"

The Powerful Trance:
When you are in a trance, you are in a different mental state. You are still awake and in control, but your emotions become incredibly focused. In this state you are more receptive to any suggestions you may receive from a Certified Hypnotherapist or that you give yourself with self-hypnosis.

Some trances are deeper than others. In a light trance, you feel more relaxed and are able to respond to simple suggestions. In a heavier trance, you can learn how not to respond to pain and even to forget what occurred in hypnosis.

Inducing a Light Trance:
The Induction Technique. The Nine Steps to Take:

1. Find a comfortable position in a dimly lit room where you won't be interrupted. The room should be neither too hot nor too cold; 71 to 73 degrees is a nice setting for the thermostat. Relax. You may want to remove your shoes and this is fine.

2. Focus on an object across the room; the corner of a picture or some flowers in a vase on a table. Anything is fine. Try to find an object that is a tad above your normal line of sight so you have to strain a bit looking up to see the object.

3. As you look at your spot, silently say to yourself:
"My eyelids are getting heavier and heavier."
"My eyelids feel as if heavy weights are pulling them down."
"Soon they will be so heavy they will close."
Repeat these three sentences for 45 seconds, approximately three times for each sentence, spoken in a slow cadence.

4. Focus on your eyelids. Soon you will feel your eyelids getting heavier. Feel this heaviness deepen with time. Let it happen. Relax and it will happen.

5. As your eyes begin to close, say to yourself:
"Relax and let go."

6. When your eyes close, take in a deep breath through your nostrils and hold that breath for 10 seconds.

7. Slowly exhale through your slightly parted lips, making a "swooshing" sound. At the same time, let your jaw drop and feel a wave of warmth and heaviness spread

from the top of your head, down your body, all the way to your toes.

8. Continue to breath slowly and smoothly. As you exhale, silently say the word "calm" or "relax" or some other relaxing word to yourself.

9. As you breathe, let feelings of relaxation deepen for another few moments and enjoy the relaxed state you are in.

After you induce a light trance, you are ready to move into a deeper state of hypnosis.

Going a Little Deeper.
The Nine Steps:

1. Take a deep breath and hold for 10 seconds.

2. Exhale slowly through your lips while you say the word "deeper" to yourself. Continue this process for several more breaths, saying the word "deeper" to yourself with every exhalation.

3. Imagine you are stepping onto a descending escalator, a slow escalator that will take you into a state of deeper relaxation.

4. As you begin your descent, silently say to yourself: "I am sinking slowly into a deeper state of relaxation."

5. As you descend, count backwards on each exhalation, from 10 to 1.

6. When you reach the bottom of the escalator, imagine you are stepping off this escalator and are now stepping onto a second descending escalator.

7. As you imagine your descent, deepen your trance with each breath, again counting backwards from 10 to 1.

8. Continue to deepen your trance until you feel you have reached a comfortable level of relaxation.

9. You may need one escalator ride or you may need several. With practice, a deeper trance will come more quickly and more easily to you.

Getting Out of The Trance

You are now in a trance. You are feeling relaxed and your mind is at peace. You can choose to remain in this relaxed state and enjoy the benefits of relaxation and calm. You can give yourself a suggestion that can extend the relaxation beyond the trance state. Here is the formula:

- Simply count backward from 5 to 1. Say to yourself beforehand:

- "When I reach 1, my eyes will open and I will feel totally awake and refreshed."

- As you count, notice your eyes may begin to flutter and begin to partially open as you approach 1.

- When you reach 1, which you say silently to yourself, your eyes will open and you will be totally awake and refreshed.

Here are three different Direct Suggestions to put you on your way to losing that excess weight. Only one Direct Suggestion is given after you have entered the hypnotic state and before you are ready to get out of the hypnotic state. When hypnosis is conducted on a different day, you can use a different Direct Suggestion.

"You now have the skills to see the circumstances and people that cause you to overeat. You accept the fact that you have control over your emotions and your eating habits, not allowing them to control you. You want to be slim and healthy and your appetite is satisfied with smaller amounts of food than you are used to. You crave healthy and nutritious foods and eating them in amounts that are necessary to reach and maintain your ideal weight."

"Your commitment to a slimmer healthier you is so deep that you are no longer tempted by unhealthy rich foods. Your commitment is so strong that it easily controls your appetite. You automatically eat the foods your body needs in the right portions. You have no desire to eat more than is necessary to maintain your health."

"As the pounds melt away, you are beginning to look and feel the way you want to look and feel; slim, trim, and fit. You feel filled with vim, vigor, and vitality. Your energy is electric. You have a new pulse on life. You enjoy life with gusto."

Here are Six Guided Imagery Ideas, two for each type of learner; three for Relaxation and three for Weight Loss. You can use them interchangeably if you desire. These Guided Imagery ideas are utilized as you silently verbalize your Direct Suggestion.

For Relaxation: (Always picture yourself as the new slimmer and trimmer you as you visualize the follows pictures).

1. Auditory:

"Hear yourself being totally relaxed from the top of your head to the tip of your toes. You can hear the calmness in your body. It's like a symphony has been induced in your body with micro-chips and with every deep breath you take, another sound-wave of calm is released with every exhalation of breath. You hear the trees swaying in the wind, but are too relaxed to move and touch them. You hear the calm music the birds are singing, but are too relaxed to join their choir. You hear your own breathing which calms you even more. You hear "calm" when you breathe in and "calm" when you breathe out; boy, does this feel calm and relaxing."

2. Visual:

"See yourself being totally relaxed from the top of your head to the tip of your toes. Your eyes feel sleepy because you have no worries. Your shoulders are totally free of any weights or burdens. You see your stomach going in and out, just like a baby who hasn't got a care in the world. Your ears see the calming music of a great classical symphony. Your toes are so relaxed they could almost dance, but they are too relaxed to get up. You see a totally 100% worry-free person and feel 100% relaxed, refreshed, and renewed; boy does this feel great."

Kinesthetic:

"Feel yourself being totally relaxed from the tip of your head to the tips of your toes. You can feel the calmness in every muscle in your body. Your head feels so light. Your shoulders feel almost weight-less. Your stomach, as you breathe slowly in and out, brings a new feeling of calm and relaxation with every breath. In is "calm" and out is "calm." Your toes feel so relaxed they could almost float away. Feel the great feeling of total, 100% relaxation with every pore of your skin; boy does this feel great."

For Weight Loss

Auditory:
"Hear yourself with the new pride you have in your new trim figure. You hear compliments wherever you go. At home, your family is filled with joy at the new you. They express their joy loudly and frequently. Your co-workers don't miss a beat and tell you how fabulous you look in your new body. The hairdresser, the tailor, the clerk at the grocery store are generous with their verbal praises of your commitment and success. You hear this loudly and clearly and it sounds great."

Visual:
"See yourself in your new body. It is trimmer, slimmer, and filled with more vigor. You step on the scale and you see that magic number that in the past years has eluded you; now, the number is a reality. You look in the mirror and you see a firm and healthy body. You see the

smile on your face that exemplifies your commitment to your success. You see your body strutting your new you in a swimsuit that says: "Look at me. I did it." See the pride in your eyes as you acknowledge you now have your vibrant health and vitality as a permanent part of your life; boy, does this look great; I look great and I feel great."

Kinesthetic:
"Feel your new body. You have places you haven't felt in years. You now uncover those glorious places with your fingertips. No rolls of fat. All you feel is smooth, slim curves in all the right places. Feel your sense of pride and accomplishment. Your commitment has paid off big time; a smaller you on the outside, but a more confident person on the inside. Now you can feel the expression; "Great things come in small packages." You are laced with energy and vitality and you can feel the energy surging through your body. It is totally awesome; boy, does this feel great."

We learn by repetition and therefore I've included a suggestion on making two different audio tapes; one for weight-loss and maintenance and the other for relaxation. You can do this on your own if you have a pleasant voice or you can engage someone who has a pleasant voice to listen to.

Use the scripts above and practice them so they feel natural and comfortable before you approach the microphone. If you want to intersperse your own words, go ahead and be creative. The idea is to tape a voice that you will enjoy listening to over and over again while you are hearing words that will reach your subconsious mind. You will be changing your eating habits and lifestyle habits as your mind listens to the words and ultimately does what it is told to do; so elementary and basic, yet so effective and life changing.

Here are The Thirteen Ingredients (The Baker's Dozen) to open the door to successful self-hypnosis:

1. Use a tape recorder that is easy to use, and speak in a slow and soothing manner.

2. Use different tones of emphasis for different areas you want to emphasize.

3. Pause 2 to 3 seconds after the word "calm" when it is used.

4. You can sit or lie down in a comfortable room where you won't be interrupted.

5. Prepare a schedule that will work for you and one that you will stick with. Your health depends on it.

6. I suggest a minimum of 3 sessions per week, although in the first week or two, 4-5 is a great way to jumpstart your motivation and determination. Later, for maintenance and the fabulous health benefits of relaxation, I suggest visiting yourself with self-hypnosis at least 2-3 times a week. You'll love the life long benefits, and might even become addicted; one of those healthy addictions, like exercising and living life with gusto.

7. Keep a journal to jot down each session and a brief description of how good it felt. This is a key component in the beginning of the weight-loss program and after many lost pounds later, it is a great incentive for other goals you may want to reach in your life where hypnosis can be quite beneficial.

8. Keep it simple, simon (KISS). A space you can call your own. A comfortable outfit to wear for each session. A consistent time several days a week where you won't be interrupted; you have a committed appointment with yourself and for yourself.

9. You deserve to improve the quality of your life, so begin today and don't delay.

10. Share your success with others when you feel comfortable doing so.

11. Be positive. Be focused on success. Be patient.

12. Enjoy the experience.

13. Let each pound that you lose, stay lost. Yet remember, that if a pound or two comes back occasionally, you know where and how to remove the excess weight. Your new found knowledge among these pages, spoken by your personal "Mind-Body-Spirit" Coach, will get you there now, and if you need a tune-up later, I'll be here for you in the future.

CHAPTER 8

▼

DIET

Diet and Maintenance.

I like choices and I want you to feel empowered to make healthy choices. I have included three different "Diet and Lifestyle" programs that can change your life. These programs are unique in the respect that they have been practiced for many years, by many people, and are centered around a balanced food program as well as an exercise program. Get ready to discard your negative thinking of deprivation and starvation. Read your "Mind-Body-Spirit" Coaches words as I present food for thought and thoughts of food in a positive and powerful environment. Open your mind to a new and exciting path to better health and greater wealth in your life. Dr. David Simon, the Medical Director of the Chopra Center and

Spa for Well Being in Carlsbad, California, whom I had the privilege of interviewing, said it best: "Good food is better than good medicine."

A few inspiring words about eating "consciously" and the positive effect this has on weight loss. Your excess weight is caused not just by what you eat, but also how you've been eating the food; carelessly or compulsively; on the run instead of sitting down; irregular meals. These behaviors make a big difference in weight loss and maintenance. They begin with bad habits. Bad habits built into the subconscious mind over time and can be changed into good habits. This process begins with "conscious awareness." Everyones body has the intelligence to know the right amount of food to eat; nature gave us hunger (versus appetite) to know the right amount to eat and when we are satisfied, the satiation reflex, it's opposite. When you go on automatic pilot and eat without "conscious awareness," then triggers (discussed in a previous chapter) can send you grabbing for food.

I am presenting thirty ingredients to help you become a mindful eater. Copy them down and post them in two or three places around your home and work or play environments. Practice them with a positive mental attitude so they become an energizing force in your Mind-Body-Spirit Roadmap to health and vitality.

The Thirty Ingredients:

1.   Eat in a settled atmosphere.

2.   Never eat when you are upset.

3.   Always sit down to eat.

4.   Reduce ice cold food and drink.

5.   Don't talk while chewing food.

6.   Eat at a moderate pace.

7.   Wait between meals before enjoying the next meal.

8.   Eat only when you feel hungry.

9.   Sip warm or room temperature water with your meals.

10.   Eat freshly cooked meals when possible.

11.   Eat cooked foods if you have a digestion problem.

12.   Do not cook with raw honey.

13. Experience the different tastes available at each meal, such as salty, sweet, pungent, astringent, and bitter.

14. Use pretty plates.

15. Set an attractive table with flowers and candles and consider some soft and soothing background music.

16. If you drink milk, make sure you drink it between your meals, and if you have digestive problems, make sure it is warm or hot milk.

17. Leave one-third to one-fourth of your stomach empty to aid your digestion.

18. Sit quietly for a few minutes after your meal.

19. Eat fresh foods suitable to your own area when possible; for example, fresh strawberries and oranges if you live in California.

20. Have your largest meal at lunch. This is the time when your digestion is best.

21. Breakfast should be your smallest meal of the day because you have been fasting for many hours and you do not want to overload your stomach.

22.   Try to eat at the same time each day when it is practical and possible.

23.   Avoid eating at night after you have had your evening meal. If you find you are a bit hungry, you might try some warm milk before going to bed.

24.   Dine alone or eat with people you genuinely care about. Tension in the air can float to tension on the inside, and your digestion will be the battleground in the end.

25.   Leave negative emotions at the front door.

26.   Wait a few moments after a meal to digest your food. Lingering is good for you and your digestion.

27.   Avoid negative self-talk. Your entire body is affected by negativity of any kind and will have negative effects on your attempts at a positive lifestyle.

28.   Savor each bite and enjoy the experience.

29.   Avoid snacking. It is far better to concentrate on your main meals then to snack between meals. You will enjoy your meals more and look forward to them.

30.   Be grateful for natures gift of food and respect it with each bite you take.

Below is a history lesson in Nutrients for your health: Here are the ingredients for a healthy eating plan that will last you a lifetime:

Fats:
There are healthy and unhealthy fats. Our body needs fat to survive and thrive. Here is the sensible way for you to see the good fats versus the bad fats in your foods.

Saturated Fats: These are the bad fats. When taken in *excess,* saturated fats raise your levels of blood cholesterol and clog your arteries. It's found mostly in animal products, such as beef, pork, chicken, milk, and other dairy products (the regular kind, not non or low fat.) The amount of fat in these foods varies widely. For example, a four ounce portion of pork tenderloin has only two grams of saturated fat versus four ounces of beef ribs, which has twelve grams of saturated fat.

The major health organizations recommend keeping your saturated fat number to less than 10% of your total calories. If you eat 2000 calories daily, that means you can get 200 of these from saturated fat because one gram of saturated fat, or fat of any kind, contains nine calories; you can eat approximately twenty-two grams of saturated fat daily.

Trans-Fats: These artery-clogging fats are as harmful to your body as saturated fats. They are created by a process that turns liquid oils into solids like margarine and shortening. Crackers, chips, cookies, pastries, certain types of breads, cereals, and peanut butter may contain trans-fats. Look for the word "hydrogenated" or "partially hydrogenated" on labels and avoid products that contain them. Be a conscious reader. Be aware and responsible for what goes into your shopping cart, onto your plate, and into your mouth.

Unsaturated Fats: These are the "good for you" fats. They are found in a variety of oils, such as canola, olive, flaxseed, sesame, sunflower, soy, safflower, and peanut oil. They are also found in foods such as flaxseed, olives, peanuts, almonds, cashews, natural peanut butter, and fatty fishes such as red salmon, mackarel, and sardines.

There are two kinds of Unsaturated Fats; Mono and Poly:

Mono-Saturated Fats:
Olive oil, canola oil, natural peanut butter, and avocados.

Poly-Saturated Fats:
Corn oil, soybean oil, and sunflower oil.

Evidence strongly suggests that mono-saturated fats may help protect against heart disease by reducing levels of LDL cholesterol (the artery clogging kind) without affecting HDL (the kind that acts as a vacuum cleaner within your bloodstream, ie. the good kind).

Major health organizations recommend keeping your total fat intake to less than 30% of your total calories (66 fat grams) if you eat a 2000 calorie diet. However, the Greek population of the 1960's ate as much as 40% fat, primarily from olive oil, and their heart disease rates were 9% lower than those of Americans. The important figure to concentrate on is the saturated fat number; keep it to less than 10% of your total calories.

Carbohydrates:

Carbohydrates are the bodys main source of fuel. 50% is an acceptable number if you exercise, and I know you will be excited and motivated to exercise after you read the upcoming chapter on exercise. The key is to favor complex carbohydrates over processed simple sugars. Complex carbohydrates have sugar molecules strung together in long chemically bonded chains. These carbo-hydrates are found in beans, whole wheat pasta, grains, and vegetables. This sugar in complex carbohydrates is absorbed slowly into your bloodstream so that your blood sugar level and energy level remain fairly constant throughout the day and you feel full for a good while.

Fiber:

The Federal Government recommends twenty to thirty grams of fiber daily. Fiber comes from whole grain products, vegetables, fruit, oats, whole wheat bread, dry beans, peas, nuts, and seeds. Be sure to eat the skin on most fruits and vegetables when applicable and always wash them properly. Here are the fabulous benefits of fiber in a varied diet; it keeps the colon healthy, your bowel movements regular, reduces cholesterol and gives you a feeling of fullness longer throughout the day.

Avoid processed Carbohydrates.

Simple carbohydrates are single or double sugar molecules. They are found in table sugar and processed foods like cakes, cookies, and colas. They also occur naturally in fruit. Simple carbohydrates, whether found in a papaya or a pop tart, are absorbed quickly, causing the amount of sugar in your blood to skyrocket and plunge soon after, leaving you feeling tired and hungry. But, there is a big difference between natural sugar in fruit and refined sugar in a candy bar. When you eat fruit such as an apple or a pear, the sugar comes packed with vitamins, minerals, water and fiber. The candy bar has few, if any redeeming qualities. The rule of thumb is to eat foods as natural as possible.

Protein:

Protein is made of amino acids that your body uses to build and repair your muscles, red blood cells, enzymes and other tissues. If you are fairly active, your goal should be .5 to .75 grams of protein per pound of body weight.

The importance of Liquids.

Over 75% of your body is made of water; even bone is more than 20%. When you don't drink enough water, your blood doesn't flow properly and your digestive track doesn't run smoothly. New research indicates drinking plenty of water can reduce the risk of breast, colon, and urinary cancers. A good recommendation is to drink eight cups of water daily and here is the math. You lose ten cups of water daily; two cups to sweating and evaporation; two cups to breathing and six cups through the water in the foods you eat. You have to make up the remaining eight cups by drinking fluids, and water is your best friend. Water is absolutely critical for the proper functioning of your organs. Keep a water bottle with you at all times; your desk at work, in your purse or briefcase and in your car. Here is another tip for a balanced fluid intake. To prevent dehydration, drink water all day long, with and between your meals. Your body and mind will thank you with clearer thinking capabilities, more focus and a balanced internal thermostat system.

Vitamin and Mineral Supplements.

The Department of Agriculture reports that 90% of the population fail to get enough magnesium, chromium, Vitamins A, B, and E, Zinc and other nutrients on a daily basis. To meet these guidelines, you would have to overdose on a specific food, over and over again. For example, research suggests Vitamin E may lower your risk of cancer and heart disease, but you would have to get that much from your diet by eating twenty-five cups of spinach or drink a tad over one cup of vegetable oil. To meet the recommended amount of Vitamin C, you would have to eat eighteen oranges. The simple answer is to eat a healthy and varied diet chosen from these pages. In addition to eating a variety of abundant fruits and vegetables with your meals, take a good multi-vitamin daily, geared toward your age and gender. The American Medical Association came out with validation for the efficacy of vitamins in 2002, by recommending that every adult take a daily vitamin supplement. Read the labels for men under and over the age of 50 and the same for women. Women should increase their amount of calcium, magnesium and Vitamin D to maintain strong bones, and everyone should try to get adequate amounts of sunshine to help the body absorb these nutrients; twenty minutes daily with proper sunscreen not only feels good but is good for your bones. One nutritionist coined it with humor, yet within a serious context, when he said: "Forget the cow. Take your dog for a twenty minute walk." If you don't have a dog, borrow one from your neighbor.

Here is your Nutritional Insurance Policy:
"Vitamins in a nutshell: A daily dose of a Baker's Dozen Vitamins."

1. Vitamin A: 5000 Units. Needed for the eyes. Found in broccoli, cantaloupe, and spinach.

The B Vitamins. Needed for the blood stream and energy.
2. Vitamin B1:   10-50 mg.   Found in chicken, garbanzo beans, and pinto beans.

3. Vitamin B2:   10-100 mg.   Found in almonds, walnuts, and low fat yogurt.

4. Vitamin B3:   20-100 mg.   Found in hazelnuts, walnuts, and sunflower seeds.

5. Vitamin B5:   10-250 mg.   Found in black beans, garbanzo beans, and lentils.

6. Vitamin B6:   50-100 mg.   Found in eggs, halibut, mackerel, and salmon.

7. Vitamin B12:   5-100 mg.   Found in yogurt and halibut.

8. Vitamin C: The key component for healthy connective tissues and your bones.

1000 mg.   Found in all citrus foods, berries such as strawberries, blueberries, boysenberries, green and yellow fruits and vegetables, and red peppers.

9. Vitamin D: Needed in combination with Calcium to strengthen your bones.

600-800 mg.   Found in capsule or tablet form. For those who live in sunny climates, the best source is the natural rays of the sun, best before 10am and after 3pm.

Calcium: Needed to build and repair healthy bones and teeth.

1200-1500 mg.   For those under 50 years of age, 1200 is your goal. For those 50 and over, your goal is 1500 mg. daily.   Found in sardines, wheat germ, beans, broccoli, spinach, tofu, almonds, walnuts, dairy products such as kefir, yogurt, cheese, and milk.

11. Magnesium: Needed to help your body absorb the Vitamin D and calcium.

Vitamin supplements provide the adequate amount. For the natural and tummy satisfying way, have a bowl of oatmeal in the morning.

12. Vitamin E: Needed to protect against free radicals destroying cells in your body.
50 units.   Found in almonds, hazelnuts, wheat germ, sweet potatoes and grains.
13. Folic Acid: Needed to repair breaks in DNA.
200 mcg.   Found in spinach, lentils, black beans, kidney beans, orange juice, chicken and avocado.

With a firm foundation of foods and their nutrients, along with your Nutritional Insurance Policy of Vitamins, I will now present three eating programs that exemplify nutritional eating and an active lifestyle.

"Mediterranean Lifestyle Diet"

The Mediterranean Diet Pyramid came out in 1992. It is ideal because it truly involves an entire lifestyle of activity and diet. It is based around the findings of the Greeks and Italians around the 1960's, when thousands of people were part of a study, many living into their 80's and 90's. At the time, their chronic disease rates were among the worlds lowest and adult life expectancy was the highest, despite limited medical resources in those regions at the time of findings.

Meat ... 3-4 times monthly

Sweets ... 1 serving weekly

Eggs ... 7 per week

Poultry ... 3-5 servings per week

Fish.... 3-5 servings per week

Cheese and yogurt ... 2 servings daily

Olive oil ... liberally and daily

Fruit ... 3-5 servings daily

Vegetables ... 3-5 servings daily

Legumes and beans ... 2-3 servings daily

Bread, pasta, rice, couscous, polenta, other whole grains and potatoes ... 7-11 servings daily

Water ... 6 glasses daily

Wine ... in moderation

Their lifestyle did and continues to include daily physical activity, mostly walking. They socialized and continue to socialize with family and friends on a daily basis. They have always had strong ties to their community. They enjoyed and continue to enjoy keeping journals and possess a positive mental attitude and a zest for life.

"The 2000 Version of The Mediterranean Diet"

In the early 2000's, the Harvard School of Public Health came out with their version of the Mediterranean Diet.

Red meat, butter, white rice and white pasta and sweets ... use sparingly.

Dairy ... 1 to 2 times daily

Fish, poultry, and eggs ... 0 to 2 times daily

Nuts and legumes ... 1 to 3 times daily

Fruits and vegetables ... 8 to 10 times daily

Whole grain foods at most meals ... daily

Plant oil, including olive, canola, corn and soy ... 2 times daily

Daily exercise is the component that gives the above foods balance and should be indulged in daily, keeping an eye on variety and enjoyment. The recommended minimum amount of exercise for health is twenty minutes daily and your goal should ultimately be thirty to forty-five minutes daily.

"The Okinawa Program"

Okinawa is located in the Southern Seas between China and Japan. A twenty-five year study was conducted with twenty-five centenarians. The results were so remarkable that National Geographic Magazine highlighted the story and the people on the cover and through the pages of one of their 2005 issues. The lifestyle of these people allows them the distinction of enjoying the longest life expectancy in the entire world!!! You should read this last sentence again; it is absolutely food for thought for a vibrant, energetic, and healthy long life. The great news is that there are no sacrifices involved. Read on and I believe you will agree with your "Mind-Body-Spirit" Coach, that by utilizing the Okinawa Program, you will have the best of both worlds; nutrients and foods to fill your body, which in turn allows your body to move with agility and longevity.

Here are the findings:

- Young arteries
- Low stress levels
- Lean and fit bodies
- Sharp minds
- Positive attitudes

Here are the lifetime determinates:

- Diet

- Regular exercise

- No smoking

- Stress management (see my chapter on stress)

- Psycho-spiritual outlook (read my forthcoming chapters)

Okinawian Proverb: "Food should nourish life. This is the best medicine."

The fourteen diet principles of the Okinawa Diet:

- Eat a variety of foods, mainly from plant sources

- Eat at least five or more servings of fruits and vegetables daily

- Eat six or more servings of grain-based foods daily. Rice is the most commonly single food eaten. They favor three different types of rice. (1) Sticky Japanese Rice. (2) Buckwheat Noodles, also called Soba Noodles. (3) Whole Wheat Noodles, also called Udon Noodles. All three types of rice can be found in your regular food markets, in addition to oriental markets

- Make complex carbohydrates the basis of the diet with more than 50% of your total calories

- Limit fat to 30% of your total calories; 15% is mono-saturates; 10% is poly-saturates; the remaining is saturated fats

- Salt intake is less than 6% daily (3 teaspoons)

- Vegetables …. 7-13 servings

- Fruits …. 2-4 servings

- Whole grains…. 7-13 servings

- Calcium foods…. 2-4 servings

- Omega 3 foods …. 1-3 servings

- Vegetable oil …. 1-2 Tablespoons

- Meat, poultry, fish and eggs…. 0-6 servings

- Omega 3 foods translate into 2 Tablespoons chopped walnuts; 3 ounces cooked fish; one egg; one Tablespoon canola oil

Dr. Makoto Suzuki in his book "Okinawa Program," elaborates on the benefits of the foods so one can actually get a birds eye view of the dynamics of healthy and natural foods. Below are his creative and powerful words:

- "Go fish" … For omega 3, found in fatty fish

- Brown rice … For long life

- Berries … For the flavonoids that are found in the dark skins of berries and are more powerful antioxidants than Vitamin C and E and more effective than aspirin at reducing inflamation

- Blueberries ... Best because they delay the onset of aging and age-related memory loss by shielding the brain cells from chemicals, plaque, or trauma

- Vitamin B and C ... Eat your B's found in broccoli, bok choy, and brussel sprouts as well as your Vitamin C, which are found in cauliflower and cabbage

- Sow your oats ... Oats prevent colon cancer

- Chew, Chew, Chew ... Chew your food thirty times before swallowing because "your stomach doesn't have teeth." Also, eating slowly prevents heartburn

- Don't kill your food with too much fire ... Lightly steam, stirfry, or broil your food

- Nuts and seeds ... Keep you young. Eat them daily to help improve your circulation and muscle tone

- Open sesame ... Use oil and sesame seeds liberally. It is a blood builder and bowel protector and may prevent cancer

- Vim and vinegar ... Apple cider vinegar promotes gastro-intestinal health by balancing the PH in your body

- Mushrooms ... The ultimate longevity food. They boost your immune system, lower the bad cholesterol, regulate your blood sugar and protect the body from cancer and virus

- Tomatoes ... The red color prevents cancer

- Olive oil ... Lowers your blood pressure

- Spice up your circulation ... Spices, such as garlic, onion, cayenne, and tumeric, have been clinically shown to prevent blood clots and improve your circulation

- Fiber ... Acts like a broom to sweep out toxins from your intestinal system

- Broccoli ... For reducing your risk of lung cancer

- Spices ... Help your digestion. Poor digestion results in gas, bloating, and fatigue. Use a variety, including dill, oregano, basil, coriander, rosemary, bay, ginger, tumeric, fennel, cardamon and others. Use them in cooking or steep them as a tea to drink after your meals

- Spinach ... Makes you strong and is good for your eyesight

- Eat low on the food chain ... The higher you go, the more toxins you eat. For example, in the ocean, the top of the food chain, are large fish like swordfish and tuna, who eat smaller fish who eat even smaller fish. At the end of the chain, the tiniest fish eat plants, such as algae and botanical plankton. Thus, the largest fish have the highest levels of poisons. For land animals, like ourselves, the best idea is to eat at the bottom of the chain; beans, legumes, fruits, nuts, seeds, and other plants

- Oils ... Essential for nerve and brain function. Oils should be eaten within three months. The best place to purchase your oil is at a health food store. Olive, walnut, flaxseed and soy are excellent oils for your health. Make sure you read the label and see "cold pressed" and store your oils in the refrigerator in dark glass containers

All three Lifestyle Programs include balance and variety. Your body will love the energy and vitality it generates and for a French flavor, may I refer to the French who coined the phrase, "A Votre Sante" ("To Your Health.")

CHAPTER 9

▼

EXERCISE

Exercise and Movement
  Five Ingredients for Fitness Success:

- Set specific realistic goals. For example: Commit to walking two to three times a week for 30 minutes each time for a short-term goal and thirty to forty-five minutes five to six times a week for your long term goal. Get your fitness tested. This pinpoints the area or areas you need to work on, such as aerobic conditioning, strength, flexibility or balance

- Dress the part. This is for safety reasons and comfort reasons, as well as motivational reasons to feel fired up about your workout

- Keep a daily exercise diary. Recording the details of how much you walked, how hard you pushed, how many repetitions you did and how you felt during your workout will make your motivation and self confidence soar

- Pace yourself. Don't do three hours of exercise the first week. Work up to this goal gradually. If you push too hard initially, especially if you have been a couch potato for a long time, you will encounter that pesky, yet real feeling of burn out

- Work out with a buddy or join a gym. You will increase your motivation and feel good about motivating others in the process of improving your own health

Five Fitness Myths Debunked ... Do not believe these Myths.

Myth #1—You must exercise for 30 consecutive minutes.

Reality—Three-10 minute sessions of exercise burn as many calories and provide nearly the same health benefits as one-30 minute session.

Myth #2—Lifting weights will turn you into a World Wrestling Federation contender.

Reality—Virtually all women and most men can't develop huge muscles without spending many hours daily at the gym lifting heavy weights.

Myth #3—If you stop exercising, your muscles will turn to fat.
Reality—They'll just shrink. Fat and muscle are two different entities; you can't turn one into the other.

Myth #4—By focusing on abdominal exercises, you can lose that beer gut.
Reality—You can't selectively zap fat off a particular part of your body.

Myth #5—Exercising during pregnancy increases the rate of miscarriages and or birth defects.
Reality—With a doctors approval, prenatal exercise is good for you and your baby. Studies show labor and delivery are easier for women who exercise during pregnancy.

Testing For Fitness.
When you embark on the world of weight training, the following tests will be invaluable for your safety, as well as your goals of gaining muscle mass and strength.
Go to a qualified fitness trainer at the gym or the YMCA or YWCA. Here are the key tests you need to take:

- Health History; you can go to your doctor and get a copy for your fitness trainer

- What's your heart rate?

- What's your blood pressure?

- How much of you is fat?

- How strong are you?

- How flexible are you?

Short Term Goals: One to three months:
Three examples:

- Bicycle 90 minutes a week for the next three months

- Take two yoga classes a week

- Use the stair-climber two times a week for 30 minutes each time

Long Term Goals: Three to six months:
Three examples:

- Drop 3% body fat in fifteen weeks

- Walk one mile in under fifteen minutes

- Drop twenty points from your cholesterol count

The Success Recipes for a Balanced Exercise Program; the 3 Winners are:

- Stretching

- Strength Training

- Aerobic

- Stretching

Stretching is the key ingredient to a flexible body; how far you can easily move your joints. As you get older, your tendons (the tissues that connect muscle to bone) begin to shorten and tighten, restricting your flexibility. Flexibility is also one of the keys to good posture.

Six Ingredients for a safe flexibility workout:

- Stretch as often as you can, preferably on a daily basis

- Move into each stretching position slowly

- Notice how much tension you feel. This should feel between mild and the edge of discomfort

- Focus on the area you are stretching

- Never, never, never bounce

- Hold each position for a few moments and take at least two breaths; never hold your breath

Your goal for your stretching program, combined with your strength training and aerobic (cardio), should be a minimum of three hours per week and some people benefit from four hours. Remember, you want balance in your macro life, as well as your micro (exercise) life.

- Aerobic Exercise (Cardio)
  Cardio means "For your heart." It strengthen your heart and lungs; it burns lots of calories.

Two Rules to follow with your Cardio exercising.

Rule #1—Warm up for five to ten minutes. For example, a runner would start off with a five or ten minute brisk walk. Warming up is very important because it increases the temperature in your muscles and tissues that connect muscles to bone (tendons) and bone to bone (ligaments). Warmer muscles and joints are looser and less likely to tear.

Rule #2—Cool down for five to ten minutes. Ease out of your workout just as you eased into it by walking or cycling lightly. The purpose of the cool-down is the opposite of the warm up; it prevents blood from pooling in one place, such as your heart.

A Cardio Recipe for good health:

A realistic goal to lower your risk of heart disease is a thirty minute work-out three times a week.

For weight loss, you need five to six work outs for a total of 45 minutes of cardio and strength training.

They can be divided; a balanced combination could be 30 minutes of cardio and 15 minutes of strength training. This should be liberally sprinkled with stretching during the course of the day.

Great activities to enjoy for your 30 minute cardio goal:

- Aerobic dance ....…......burns 342 calories
- Basketball ....…......burns 282 calories
- Bicycling (15 mph) ......….........burns 354 calories
- Boxing ....……......burns 330 calories
- Golf ....burns 174 calories
- Karate ....….......burns 150 calories
- Running (10 mph) ....….............burns 265 calories
- Tennis (singles) ....…...burns 262 calories
- Walking (15 mph with hills) .....burns 279 calories
- Strength Training
  Here are five good reasons to have a strength training program.
- Staying young for life. People who don't exercise lose 30 to 40% of their strength by the age of 65
- Keeping your bones healthy. By the age of 35, most people, men and women, begin to lose 1/2 to 1% of their bone each year. Strength training alone can't stop bone loss, but it can play a big role, along with calcium, Vitamin D, and aerobic exer-

cising such as walking or any other weight-bearing exercise

- Preventing injuries. When your muscles are strong, you are less prone to injury. You will have a better sense of balance

- Looking better. Weight training firms, builds, and shapes your muscles. It also improves your posture

- Speeding up metabolism. Dieting alone tends to cause a loss in muscle as well as fat. If you can lift weights while cutting caloric intake, you can preserve muscle and maintain metabolism while you are losing fat

The Rules of Strength Training:

Remember that lifting weight is an art, not a science, so follow these rules:

- Get your doctors blessings

- Train at a gym with proper instruction from a qualified fitness instructor

- Begin slowly; Rome wasn't built in a day

- Don't work out two consecutive days in a row

- Have fun, enjoy, and grow in your muscle mass as well as in your mental and physical health

The secret of aging slowly with good health, is fitness combined with a healthy eating program. The Journal of Gerontology recently released a study showing people over the age of sixty train just as hard as younger people and derive the same benefits. Great news for Baby Boomers and those in their Golden Years.

Ten Great Benefits of a Fitness Program:

- You have more energy
- You experience less depression and anxiety
- You have an easier time losing weight
- There is an increase in bone density: you build muscle strength and slow muscle deterioration that comes with age
- Exercise reduces lower back pain
- You cut the risk of heart disease, arthritis, diabetes, dementia, and colon cancer
- There is an improvement in your balance
- You feel younger
- Your mind is more alert
- You can lower your blood pressure

Some more ideas to consider regarding your exercise program. Have fun with exercise. Think about exercise the way you did as a kid; it was fun. You would go outside to be in the fresh air and run around the baseball field. Guys would throw balls in the hoops with their dad after dinner or on the weekend and girls would play hop-scotch with their friends. Who didn't love playing hide-and-go seek. Have the same positive mental attitude about exercise as an adult. Trust me when I tell you that exercise should be coined as the new eight letter word that means vibrant health, happiness, and longevity. It will make you feel great on the inside and look slimmer and trimmer on the outside, and this is a true win-win situation.

CHAPTER 10

▼

WISDOM OF THE AGES

The Holistic approach to permanent weight loss and maintenance has a healthy dose of spirituality in the preceding pages.

In this chapter, I have included words passed down through the ages that continue to inspire and motivate people from all backgrounds and cultures in our modern life. I hope you read them often and enjoy their motivating and inspiring words.

A 13th Century Poem by Rumi:
You were born with potential
You were born with goodness and truth
You were born with ideas and dreams
You were born with greatness

You were born with wings
You were not meant for crawling, so don't
You have wings
Learn to use them and fly.

An Old Chinese Poem by Chang-Tze:
"That which fills the Universe I regard as my body, and that which directs the Universe I see as my own Nature."

Mother Teresa spoke these words:
"Follow your heart without asking if it's o.k. to do so."

"Spread love wherever you go, first in your own house."

"Yesterday is gone. Tomorrow hasn't arrived. Begin it today."

Aristotle said:
"In all things of nature there is something of the marvelous."

An Old Okinawan Proverb:
"One cannot live in the world without the support of others."

Rabbi Nachman of Breslov wrote:
"As often as you can take a trip out to the fields to pray and all the grass will join you.

They will enter your prayers and give you strength to sing praises to G-D."

Buddha is responsible for these words of wisdom
"Wherever you live is your temple if you treat it like one."

"Our body is precious. It is a vehicle for awakening. Treat it with care."

A verse From Ancient Rig VEDA entitled "The Eternal Song."

"Although my spirit may wander the four corners of the earth
Let it come back to me again so that I may live and journey here.

Although my spirit may go far away over the sea
Let it come back to me again so that I may live and journey here.

Although my spirit may go far away to visit the sun and the dawn
Let it come back to me again so that I may live and journey here.

Although my spirit may wander over the lofty mountains
Let it come back to me so that I may live and journey here.

Although my spirit may go far away into all forms that live and move

Let it come back to me so that I may live and journey here.

Although my spirit may wander in the valley of Death
Let it come back to me so that I may journey here."

The most profound words ever spoken. Read these words often. Embrace them. I guarantee you the world will never be the same again:

"Everything that I see is a Miracle. Everything I touch is a Miracle." Thirteen words, just like my Thirteen Baker's Dozen, can transform your life. The number thirteen will forever been seen as a magic number, instead of the old negative thinking of associating thirteen with bad luck. Thirteen marvelous and miraculous words to be read over and over again, until you feel the power and energy of these words, and believe that the Creator is speaking to you. As the Jewish Words "La Chaim" translate into "To Life," so can these words translate into the very essence of Life. So I will end this chapter with this toast, "La Chaim, To Life," your new life as a healthier and happier person, the person you were meant to be, can be, and will be when you embrace the Thirteen Chapters you now hold in your hands and will soon hold in your heart.

CHAPTER 11

▼

THE SPIRIT WITHIN

I now come to the last facet of the "Mind, Body, and Spirit" Trio for true holistic success, health and well being, physically and mentally. This chapter deals with our positive mental attitude about oneself; our spirit. It is an attitude that makes our eyes sparkle, our hearts pound with happiness; our thoughts reaching out to all mankind; creatures large and small; the galaxies of the Universe; the moon and the stars and the sun with one true message; "I love and embrace you all."

Here is a five ingredient recipe for developing a positive mental attitude. Mix it with gusto and drink it daily in whatever portion you desire. It won't bring on excess weight; rather, it will bring on inner and outer joy and happiness that will add years, not weight, to your life.

- Acknowledge that every adversity, sorrow or defeat, whether or not you caused it to happen, contains the seed of an equivalent benefit which you can nurture into a blessing that soars above the disaster it brought

- Learn to close the door of your mind on all failures of your past

- Find the habit of saying or doing something each and every day that will make someone else feel better via the telephone, post cards or a simple act of kindness

- Attune your mind to attract the things and situations you desire by expressing in a daily prayer your gratitude for what you already have

- Acknowledge that love is the best food for your body and soul. Love changes your entire body chemistry and conditions it for the expression of a positive mental attitude. The best way to receive love is to give it away and you can't give away something that you don't already have

Enthusiasm is a first cousin to your positive mental attitude. Your positive mental attitude, as you progress toward success, is the fuel that drives things forward. Enthusiasm is power. With faith, it can transform adversity, failure and temporary defeat into unstoppable action.

Here are the five benefits of Enthusiasm. As you develop enthusiasm, you will:

- Increase the intensity of your thinking and imagination
- Build your personal initiative
- Strengthen your mental and physical health
- Gain self confidence
- Spread your enthusiasm with others

Remember that life is never static. Our bodies and cells and skin renew themselves continuously and we must constantly renew our mind with positive thoughts. You have the power of your mind to make choices. Every moment of life is a new beginning; a gift; a present to open and use and share. What we think about ourselves becomes our truth. We are creating our experiences by our thoughts and our feelings.

The thoughts we think and the words we speak create our experiences. Self love and self acceptance are the main ingredients to positive change in every area of our life.

Plant your seeds of success right now. Think of a rose bush. A healthy plant can have many roses on it. In order to get a rose bush with all those roses on it, you need to begin with a small dried seed. That seed doesn't look like a rose; it looks like a seed. Now, let's say you plant this seed in healthy soil and you water it and let the sun shine on it daily. When the first bud comes up, you don't say, "That's not a rose bush." You look at it and say, "Oh boy, it's starting to grow." Over time, you continue to water it, give it lots of sunshine and nourishing food and pull away the weeds and bugs and pests. In time, you'll have a beautiful rose bush and it all began with one seed.

The same occurs with creating a new experience. The soil you plant is in your subconscious mind. The seed is the new affirmation, for example, "I am slim, trim, and fit." The whole new experience is in this tiny seed. You water it with affirmations, for example, "I love eating healthy foods." "I love exercising my strong body." "I love feeling energized and empowered." You let the sunshine of positive thoughts beam on it. You weed the garden by pulling out any negative thoughts that may crop up. And when you first see the tiniest evidence of success, you don't stomp on it and say; "That's not enough. I wanted to lose 10 pounds this week, not 2 pounds." Instead, you look at this first breakthrough and exclaim with delight; "Oh boy, I lost weight. It's working." Then you watch yourself grow mentally and emotionally as you lose more weight physically, and experience what true success feels like. That's the spirit within you.

CHAPTER 12

▼

SPIRITUALITY

The word spirit means "breath" in its origins. Spirit pertains to the breath of life. When Aristotle spoke about spirit or soul, he meant that by virtue of which an organism is alive. When we refer to a person as being "high spirited," we mean "full of life." When we speak of a persons spirit being broken, we mean that persons will to live self-assertively has been extinguished; the life force has been snuffed out of him or her.

Today, "spirit" connotes "the life force" as manifested in consciousness. "Spirituality" pertains to "consciousness" and to the needs of consciousness. Think of spirituality as being an intangible. A spiritual person is experiencing his reality, not a tangible object. Whereas religion is centered on rituals and rules, spirituality is how one lives and how one experiences life.

Western and Eastern spiritual disciplines can work as a team for an explosive and powerful self-awareness consciousness. More and more, Westerners are exploring meditation and similar deep relaxation techniques and discovering the benefits as a path to self-understanding, enhanced creativity, a deeper appreciation of what is important in life, and the experience of greater peace, calm, and serenity.

In his book "Perfect Health," Dr. Deepak Chopra writes about the immense power of the mind and spirituality affecting our lives. Ayurveda, the ancient practice which unites the Mind-Body-Spirit Trio, that goes back thousands of years, addresses how our lives can be influenced, shaped, extended, and ultimately controlled when we allow spirituality to infuse our Body-Mind connection. He professes that the mind exerts the deepest influence on the body, and freedom from sickness depends upon contacting our own awareness, bringing it into balance and then extending that balance to the body.

This state of balanced awareness, more than any kind of physical immunity, creates a higher state of health. Over the past fifteen years, Dr. Chopra and his highly trained colleagues at The Chopra Center and Spa for Well Being in Carlsbad, California, have developed a modernized system of Ayurveda that integrates truths of this ancient approach with the most advanced insights of modern science. Dr. Chopra and his staff have treated more than 10,000 patients, blending Ayurveda and Western Medicine, bringing together ancient wisdom and modern science, and the two have proved completely compatible and successful. The patients are asked to look inward to their spiritual side and this is complemented with patient physicals and objective tests to create a life-style plan personalized for each individual patient. The results have been nothing short of miraculous.

Another dynamic illustration of spirituality in healing took the medical community by surprise in the 1980's. Dr. Dean Ornish, a San Fransisco Cardiologist, proved that forty advanced heart patients could actually shrink fatty plaque deposits that were progressively blocking their arteries. As their arteries were beginning to open, fresh oxygen started reaching their hearts, thus relieving frightening chest pains and reducing their risk of having fatal coronaries.

Rather than relying on drugs or surgery to unblock their arteries, the patients used meditation for stress reduction, yoga exercises, and a vegetarian diet.

The Insurance Industry was also taken by surprise, and following this incredible study, proceeded to pay for an eight-week program lead by Dr. Ornish, saving thousands and thousands of dollars that would have gone to the surgeons and hospitals and drug companies. The program was so successful in Northern California that

Dr. Ornish went to Southern California, and with his mentorship taught the Medical Staff at Scripts in La Jolla about the program. There is currently an Integrative Medicine Department at Scripts which teaches the disciplines of the Ornish Program, which includes yoga, meditation, exercise, healthy food choices and preparation, and lifestyle habits liberally laced with the power of a positive mental attitude.

Living consciously is an act of love for ones own positive possibilities. It is an act of commitment to ones values as a person and to the importance of ones life. It is not a duty we owe others. It is a responsibility we owe to ourselves. It is an act of commitment to our values and the importance of our life.

You owe it to yourself to read and reread all the chapters of this book utilizing the infinite power of the "Mind-Body-Spirit" Holistic Approach to reach your dreams and goals of a healthier you. Digest the positive ingredients throughout the pages. Go forward with a positive mental attitude, passion and enthusiasm for the new you, a lighter (in pounds) you and a more vibrant (in spirit) you. Maintain a new mindset that sings "I can," and you will see, feel, taste, touch, and smell the new you. You can do it. Your "Mind-Body-Spirit" Coach knows that you can do it, and now, so do you. Don't put off today what you can do today. Live and thrive in the moment. Live in the present because life is a present. Open it up and enjoy it with all of your heart and soul and share it with others!

Original Inspirational Poems by Dr. Shana Schenker:

Poem #1
Hark! I hear a voice. It must be me. Who else could it be.
The sound is bright all through the night. It lets me know I'm in control.
I choose to be a slim new me. My body and mind have found the time to work together like birds of a feather.
I see the light with all my might. I am in control, don't you just know.
It's me, oh gee I thank you naturally. It feels so great to have found my faith.
I'll stay this way forever and a day. I feel so good. I look so fine. The prize is health. It feels divine.
I hope you see it's a brand new me. I hope you feel I made the deal to be a winner being so much thinner.

Poem #2
Do you love a fatty, I'll bet you don't. The laughs can be mean like a big bad dream. People stare, they just don't care. They keep on starring. If only I could hide, anywhere, every time.
You know you shouldn't take one more bite. But your will turns around as simply as it rebounds. You some-

times eat till you drop. You know you just can't fake it till you make it.

Your will is too weak but who do you seek. You need a plan and you need it now, or else one day you will look like a clown.

You ask for assistance but you come against resistance because your mind and body just seem to frown.

You need to have the spiritual side, to have the success you desire and admire.

I'm here to tell you it can be done. Take each day, add a little play. Stop, look, and listen, because this is your mission.

You can succeed, have no fear. You'll look as good up front as you do from the rear.

Poem #3

Good luck to you it's really true. The past is past and the present has a clue.

It's called faith. It's called hope. It's called "I can see." The truth goes deep, very deep within me.

Grab your pen, your paper too. Cause I got the tools that are really quite cool. They don't cost money, tears, or sweat. They take an investment of all the rest. By that I mean a clear picture of the figure you want, desire, and admire.

What you need dear friend I tell you now, is strength, courage, and a burning desire. With an attitude of faith and an inner picture of you slim and strong so you can't go wrong.

So see it right now from this moment on, and you'll create the figure of your desire, I promise others will admire.

Poem #4

You in the mirror, what do you see? I'll bet it's fat; how pretty can that be!

You tried will power and that didn't work. Quite frankly my friend, you must feel like a jerk.

They say you're smart, but I don't know. If you were, you'd be healthy and slim like me. I know the recipe, it's clear, it is. I'll share with you right now so you'll stop looking like a clown.

I take my Body, Spirit, and Mind and treat them in kind. All working together like birds of a feather. Each day I see as vividly as can be, the figure I want with all my might and never keep this out of my sight.

I say with my voice what I want in my life, a slim new me, yes it truly can be. I repeat 5 times all through the day; "I'm successful in each and every way."

Combine this with patience, a smile, a self-hug, and the miracle will be a slim, healthy new me.

Good luck, dear friend, I truly know, you have the power and the tools to make miracles grow.

Poem #5

I'll be brief, I'll say it right. You can be and see, if you'll just believe me.

It's really simple, right from the start. You need a plan, so get on your mark.

Set the date, set it in your mind. You are really neat, you're one of a kind.

If you want to lose the weight for good, don't say I should, or won't, or would.

Dream big, set the date and make it important to you, and then your mind and body will deliver the goods.

The great news, my friend, is I'm here for you. Your "Mental Coach" with a Capital "C," it was absolutely meant to be.

So let's begin right now, not a minute too soon. We're shooting for the moon and we'll arrive before high noon.

Say "I can" "I really can," "I believe in me," "I believe, you see." My ultimate goal is fabulous health and when I attain this goal, I'll have fabulous wealth!

CHAPTER 13

▼

SMILE

Ending and Beginning with a Smile.

This final chapter is an ending and a beginning and I want you to finish the last page with a smile and a positive mental attitude and a passion for success.

Thirty original ingredients to make you feel like a kid. Practice and enjoy them often with gusto and with passion.

- Smile
- Sing
- Yoddel
- Watch a sunset
- Watch a sunrise

- Play hopscotch
- Plant a seed and water it and watch it grow
- Write a poem
- Write a letter to someone in the hospital and take it to them
- Play jacks
- Paint with your fingers
- Listen to birds sing
- Whistle
- Take a picture and send it to a friend
- Dance a jig, fox trot, or polka
- Give something to a friend or stranger
- Begin a diary
- Learn five lines of a foreign language
- Sign up for a fun class and take action
- Call a friend and say: "I love you and I'm happy you're alive."
- Count your blessings
- Doodle and daydream
- Pet a rock or a tree
- Make a scrapbook

- Take crayons and paper and go to town
- Mold a sculpture with clay
- Make pipe cleaner figures
- Blow up 5 balloons and give them away
- Bake cookies and have a bake sale and donate the money to charity
- Read the comic strips

Twenty Original Positive Affirmations. Write them on a 3x5 card. Carry them with you always. Read them. Say them. Shout them to the Universe. There are no rules, no gates, only positive words to internalize so that your mind can see and believe and allow you to achieve.

- "My tree of life has all the fruits I need to succeed"
- "He who has doubts loses the power to succeed"
- "Walk in faith and run with success"
- "I eat each meal with a conscious mindset"
- "I choose to be the best that I can be"
- "Stand tall and be tall. Believe and conceive and achieve"
- "I'm as strong as an oak tree"
- "I'm as courageous as a tiger"

- "Success begins now and can last a lifetime"
- "I am a winner, oh yea"
- "I love my new body"
- "I eat slowly and savor each bite"
- "I feel slim and trim and vibrant"
- "I am special, whole and complete"
- "I am a poster child for success"
- "The path of success beings in my mind"
- "The best role model is my body, mind, and spirit"
- "Only I can achieve the real me"
- "I declare I am delighted I am slim and trim"
- "I am the picture of vibrant health and vitality"

Twenty Original Visualizations . Picture in your mind the new you, before you become the new you. You will be trying on the new you for size and get the joy and happiness of a trimmer and slimmer you, before you are even ready to get rid of the old clothes and buy a new wardrobe, because the fat clothes swim on your new svelt and tailored body. See yourself in the following 20 pictures as if you have already reached your weight loss goal, 20, 30, 50 pounds lighter, whatever your weight loss goal is. You can add sounds and aromas to enhance the experience, such as perfume on the new wardrobe or the positive exclamations of people seeing the new you at a cocktail party; be creative because you're the producer and the director.

- In yoga class
- At a cocktail party
- At the tailors being fitted for a new wardrobe
- At a picnic in shorts and a T shirt
- In your new biking outfit
- At a 5 star restaurant, dressed to impress
- On a cruise ship at the Captains Table
- At the gym in your new sleek exercise outfit
- On the mountain top in your new ski gear
- In front of a mirror in your birthday suit
- On a sailboat in shorts, shirt, and cap
- At the zoo in a tight pair of jeans and a great new camp shirt
- At a country inn picking apples in a summer midriff bearing outfit
- On the tennis court in tennis shorts and shoes
- At your high school reunion dressed to the nines
- On stage accepting an award for your success at your new weight

- In an English Riding Outfit
- At the doctors office with your new trim body
- Looking at the scale with your ideal weight in numbers
- Walking along a country road feeling fit and fabulous

Bibliography

Atreya. Perfect Balance: Nutrition For Body, Mind and Soul. New York. Penquin Putnum, 2001.

Balch, James F., and Phyllis A Bauch. Prescription For Nutritious Healing. New York. Avery Publishing Group, 1999.

Baptiste, Sherrie and Megan Scott. Yoga with Weights. Indiana. Wiley Publishing, 2006.

Borek, Carmia. Maximize Your Health Span With Antioxidants. New Cannan, Ct Keats Publishing, 1995.

Braden, Nathaniel. The Art of Living Consciously. New York. Fireside, 1997.

Carnegie, Dale. How To Win Friends And Influence People. New York. Simon and Schuster, 1936.

Chopra, Deepak. Ageless Body, Timeless Mind: The Quantum Alternative To Growing Old. New York. Harmony, 1994.

-. Grow Younger, Live Longer. Ten Steps To Reverse Aging. New York. Three Rivers Press, 2002.

-. Perfect Health. New York. Three Rivers Press, 1991.

-.The Book Of Secrets: Unlocking The Hidden Dimensions Of Your Life. New York. Harmony, 2004.

Dyer, Wayne. The Power Of Intension. U.S.A. Hay House, 2004.

Egoscue, Pete. Pain Free. New York. Random House, 2000.

Elkin, Allen. Stress Management. New York. Wiley Publishing, 1999.

Gaia. The Essential Massage Book. London, 2005.

Haas, Elson M. Staying Healthy With Nutrition. Berkeley, CA. Celestial Arts, 1981.

Hadley, Josie and Carol Staudacher. Hypnosis For Change. Canada. Rainforest Books, 1996.

Hay, Louise. You Can Heal Your Life. U.S.A. Hay House, 1999.

Heller, Barbara. 365 Ways to Relax Mind, Body, and Soul. Mass. Storey Publishing, 2000.

Hill, Napolean. Think and Grow Rich. New York. Faucet Books, 1937.

-.Napolean Hills Keys to Success. New York. Plumb, 1997.

Inlander, Charles B. and Marie Hodge. 100 Ways to Live to 100. Allentown, PA. Peoples Medical Society, 1992.

McGraw, Phillip C. Self Matters: Creating Your Life From The Inside Out. Free Press. New York, 2003.

Mindell, Earl. Earl Mindells Anti-Aging Bible. New York. Fireside, 1996.

Nelson, Miriam. Strong Women, Stay Young. England. Penguin Books, 1997.

Osteen, Joel. Your Best Life Now. Time Warner, 2004.

Perricone, Nicholas. The Perricone Prescription. New York. Harper Collins, 2004.

-.The Perricone Promise. New York. Harper Collins, 2000.

Sears, Barry. The Anti-Aging Zone. New York. Regan Books, 1998.

Smolensky, Michael and Lynne Lamberg. The Body Clock Guide To Better Health. New York. Henry Holt and Company, 2000.

Teresa, Mother. The Joy Of Loving. India. Penquin Books, 1997.

Tourles, Stephanie. 365 Way To Energize Mind, Body, and Soul. Mass. Storey Publishing, 2000.

Weil, Andrew T. Eating Well For Optimal Health. New York. Perrenial Currents, 2001.

-.8 Weeks To Optimal Health. New York. Ballantine Books, 1998.

-.Healthy Aging. New York. Harmony, 2006.

-.Natural Health, Natural Medicine. Houghton Miffin, 2004.

-.Perfect Health: The Complete Mind Body Guide. New York. Harmony, 2001.

Wilcox, Bradley and Craig Wilcox and Makoto Suzuki. The Okinawa Program, 2001.

Zigler, Zig. Get Motivated. Better Than Good. California. Integrity Publishing, 2006.

Resources

Ask DRMAO.Com-www.askdrmao.com. Tips For Living A Long, Healthy Life. Center for Mind-Body Medicine. www.cmbm.org.

The Chopra Center and Spa. www.chopra.com. Founded by Dr. Deepak Chopra. Integrating allopathic and Indian Ayurvedic Medicine. 2013 Costa Del Mar Road. Carlsbad, CA. 92009.

Gerontology Research Group For Longevity Research. P.O. Box 905. Santa Clarita, CA. 91380-9005. www.grg.org.

Healing People Network. www.healingpeople.com. 906 E. Verdugo Road. Burbank, CA 91501.

Weil Lifestyle LLC. www.drweil.com. A website for Healthy Living based on Integrative Medicine.

Success Trak Enterprises. Dr. Bruce E. Kaloski, Chancellor and founder. Classes, Degree Programs, Seminars on Success. 1-888-437-5256.

978-0-595-46340-4
0-595-46340-1